Changing Values
in Medicine

Changing Values
in Medicine

Edited by
Eric J. Cassell, M.D.
and
Mark Siegler, M.D.

Papers delivered at the Conference on Changing Values in Medicine,
Cornell University Medical College, New York City,
November 11-13, 1979

University Publications of America, Inc.

This book is dedicated to Otto Guttentag.
Virtually alone he explored the philosophical basis of medical
practice and the role of the physician for decades before others
began to follow. We honor his work, we honor his understanding,
and we honor his example.

Library of Congress Cataloging in Publication Data

Conference on Changing Values in Medicine (1979 :
    Cornell University Medical College)
    Changing values in medicine.

    "Papers delivered at the Conference on Changing
Values in Medicine, Cornell University Medical
College, New York City, November 11–13, 1979."
    Includes bibliographies and index.
    1. Medicine—Philosophy—Congresses.   2. Physician
and patient—Congresses.   3. Humanistic psychology—
Congresses.   I. Cassell, Eric J., 1928– .
II. Siegler, Mark, 1941–   .   III. Title.   [DNLM:
1. Philosophy, Medical—congresses.   2. Physician-
Patient Relations—congresses.   W 61 C748c 1979]
R723.C664   1979   610'.1   85-10033
ISBN 0-89093-574-2
ISBN 0-89093-563-7 (pbk.)

Printed in the United States of America

Contents

Acknowledgements

The papers in this volume were presented at the conference entitled "Changing Values in Medicine" held in New York City on November 11-13, 1979, under the auspices of the Cornell University Medical College. Dean Theodore Cooper was a source not only of encouragement, but of start-up funds during a period of great budgetary constraint. His commitment helped insure a successful conference.

Generous funding for the conference and for the preparation of this volume was provided by the National Science Foundation Program for Ethics and Values in Science and Technology (NSF/EVIST). Dr. William Blanpied, then director of the program, provided more than the usual guidance and support in the preparation of the proposal, and we happily acknowledge his help.

The Conference on Changing Values in Medicine was meant to be a cohesive statement about what problems would have to be solved as medicine turned its attention away from an exclusive concern with disease and began to focus on the sick person as both the object and subject of medical care. As is widely known, it is often difficult for a large number of participants to remain centered on the same topic. We think we have been most fortunate in that regard and acknowledge our debt to our contributors. But we owe an even greater debt to Dr. Vivien Shelanski, because without her expertise as both an editor and philosopher we would truly have floundered in the task of trying to create a volume whose many voices spoke to one vital and central issue—the future of medicine.

Finally, we express our gratitude to the contributors to this volume, who generously granted us permission to publish their articles. Thanks are also due the National Humanities Center, Research Triangle Park, North Carolina, for allowing us to publish Otto E. Guttentag's "The Attending Physician as a Central Figure," which was presented there in a modified version during a conference entitled "The Humanities and the Professor of Medicine," April 16-17, 1982, and later published as part of the conference proceedings.

Contributors

MAX BLACK, Ph.D., Litt.D.
Susan Linn Sage Professor of Philosophy and Humane Studies
Senior Member, The Cornell Program for Science, Technology
   and Society
Cornell University

ERIC J. CASSELL, M.D.
Clinical Professor of Public Health
Director, The Cornell Program for the Study of Ethics and
   Values in Medicine
Cornell University Medical College

JAMES F. CHILDRESS, Ph.D.
Commonwealth Professor of Religious Studies
Professor of Medical Education
University of Virginia

H. TRISTRAM ENGELHARDT, JR., M.D., Ph.D.
Member of the Center for Ethics, Medicine and Public Issues
Professor in Departments of Medicine and Community Medicine
Baylor College of Medicine
Professor of Philosophy, Rice University

OTTO E. GUTTENTAG, M.D.
Samuel Hahnemann Professor of Medical Philosophy Emeritus
University of California, School of Medicine at San Francisco

JOHN LADD, Ph.D.
Professor of Philosophy
Chairman, Program for Biomedical Ethics
Brown University

PEDRO LAÍN ENTRALGO, M.D.
Professor of the History of Medicine
University of Madrid

ALASDAIR MACINTYRE, M.A.
W. Alton Jones Distinguished Professor of Philosophy
Vanderbilt University

ERNAN MCMULLIN, Ph.D.
O'Hara Professor of Philosophy
Director, Program for History and Philosophy of Science
Notre Dame University

EDMUND D. PELLEGRINO, M.D.
Director of the Joseph and Rose Kennedy Institute of Ethics
John Carroll Professor of Medicine and Medical Humanities
Georgetown University

STANLEY J. REISER, M.D., Ph.D.
The Griff T. Ross Professor of Humanities and Technology in
    Health Care
University of Texas Health Science Center at Houston

KENNETH F. SCHAFFNER, Ph.D.
Professor of History and Philosophy of Science
Professor of Philosophy
Adjunct Professor of Medicine
Co-chairman, University Health Center's Program for
    Human Values in Health Care
University of Pittsburgh

MARK SIEGLER, M.D.
Associate Professor in the Department of Medicine
Chief, Section of General Internal Medicine
Director, Center for Clinical Medical Ethics
University of Chicago, Pritzker School of Medicine

STEPHEN TOULMIN, Ph.D.
Professor in the Committee on Social Thought
Professor in the Department of Philosophy
Professor in the Divinity School
University of Chicago

Introduction:
Understanding the Future of Medicine

Eric J. Cassell and Mark Siegler

THE PATHS TO THE PRESENT

This book comes at a turning point in the history of medicine. It is a time, we believe, when the profession has begun to direct its attention away from an almost exclusive concern with the body and is again focusing on the sick person.

The history of medicine is a story of changing customs and costumes, instruments and methods, explanations and theories. Throughout runs the common thread of attempts to understand what makes people sick and through that understanding to make them well again. We titled this book *Changing Values in Medicine,* but a better name might have been *Enduring Values in Medicine,* for no sickness can be known apart from an appreciation of both the body and the person. It is strange that it should ever have seemed otherwise. Yet present-day disease concepts, despite their obvious utility, are conspicuous for their impersonality.

How medicine came to where it is now, and how it was ever possible to forget that sickness always involves more than only the body, is in itself instructive. The history of medicine is often written as the story of a steady and determined growth of knowledge about human biology and disease, as if the development of anatomy, physiology, biochemistry, pathology, and pathophysiology have all led inexorably to our present scientific mastery. According to that scenario, we are now in our finest hour and on the verge of even greater mastery. Some caution is necessary, because in every era commentators on medicine have spoken of the brilliant advances of their time, often forgetting that the same praises were sung about medicine in other periods which, in retrospect, seem particularly sterile.

1

The view of medical history as a steady progression is not only inaccurate, but also not very interesting. It is vastly more exciting and productive to conceive of medical history as a series of twists and turns, as excesses and droughts along an uncertain road (if that implication of directionality is even a useful metaphor), profoundly influenced by prevailing philosophies and cultures. Medicine is always a part of its contemporary world, both shaping and being shaped by that world. But its goal—the relief of sickness—has always been the same. And that goal has always been elusive.

When one of us (EJC) graduated from medical school in 1954, excitement over burgeoning therapeutic effectiveness was everywhere. People really spoke about stamping out disease! As unbelievable as it may seem, EJC was really concerned that everything would be cured and that no interesting diseases would remain. Of course, it turned out that solving some problems (primarily the big-name infectious diseases) merely allowed new and unsolvable problems to take the place of the old ones. The goal of providing adequate care for the sick is elusive precisely because of the ever-changing face of illness and the inevitable inadequacy of the physician's knowledge.

In the world of today's doctors, the patients are older, their diseases are often incurable, and society is undergoing some profound changes whose nature is not clear but whose effects are widespread. The public demands a more personal medical care governed by ethical strictures undreamed of a decade ago, care in which the patient is seen as a full and knowledgeable partner. At the same time, patients are suspicious of physicians and technology even while taking the effectiveness of both for granted. The paradoxes are numerous and discouraging to contemplate. How did we get here, and where is medicine going?

The present era of medicine started somewhat more than 150 years ago when the concept of disease as we know it came into being. Before the nineteenth century, patients presented themselves to physicians much as they do today—"dropsied and asthma'd and joint racking rheum'd." But physicians looking at those patients did not see sodium retention, small airway obstruction, or synovitis. Nor did they see rheumatic valvular disease, chronic obstructive pulmonary disease, or rheumatoid arthritis. They observed only the symptoms that could be heard or seen. To say that is merely to point to the truism that you cannot see what you do not know. Two factors impaired the ability of doctors to see beyond the obvious. First, they were overwhelmed by competing theories of how nature worked. Iatrochemists, vitalists, mechanists, and others offered different explanations of the operation of the body; proponents of each position were able to see only those facts that supported their own viewpoints. (Pres-

ent-day schools of psychology are similar.) Second, there was no cohesive nosology, or classification of disease, that could organize the
phenomena of sickness out of the chaos of endless symptom manifestations and theoretical speculation.

Around the middle of the eighteenth century, Cullen in Edinburgh
and Sauvages in Paris, among others, developed disease classifications
based on symptoms alone. In Sauvages's classification there were 2,400
"diseases"—including 18 kinds of angina, 19 kinds of asthma, 20 of
pleurodynia, 13 of cardialgia, 20 of phthisis, and so on (Faber 1923).
While those classifications were clumsy, they did represent a return
to the actual phenomena of illness as a basis for the actions of
physicians, a return to the bedside (in current jargon) and away from
theoretical speculation. But as important as that empiricism was, it
still lacked systematic guidance. The system that gave force to empirical
methods and brought medicine out of chaos was the modern
classification of disease.

The rise of modern nosologies, the classifications of disease that
we use today, is detailed in a wonderful book, *Nosology*, by Knud
Faber (1923). It is difficult to imagine the extent of the revolution
in medicine that started in Paris in the beginning of the nineteenth
century. At a lecture given recently by one of us, a student wondered
aloud what physicians of 1815 saw when they looked at tuberculosis.
The one thing they did not see was tuberculosis, because it had not
yet been invented! They may have seen the pthisis in the lung, scrofula
in the lymph nodes of the neck, kyphosis from a cold abcess of the
spine, or any one of a number of other diverse afflictions, but not
tuberculosis.

The brilliance of René Laënnec's contribution to medical progress
was that he made it clear that all these things were but different
manifestations of the same disease. He made that contribution by tying
together what he saw in the living patient with what he saw at the
autopsy, and by adding the essential element of physical examination.
This is what we today call clinicopathological correlation. Why have
we used the term *invent* rather than *discover*? We have done so to
emphasize that when Laënnec brought the various organ manifestations of tuberculosis together under one rubric, he did not merely
uncover a truth that had been lying there all along, like finding a
new species of violet in the forest; rather, he made a major conceptual
leap forward. It might have been possible to organize the reality that
turned out to be tuberculosis in another way entirely. For example,
the various presentations that we call tuberculosis, or the other afflictions presently known to be infectious, could have been viewed
as diseases of malnutrition or social status, and in such a conception
diseases would have included manifestations of the social being as

well as the body. Such disease constructions, while pointing to one set of causes, might have precluded the discovery of the mycobacterium. In fact, along with the concept of disease that developed in those years of ferment in Paris came the belief that for each disease there was a specific etiology. The revolution that started in the early 1800s with the concept of disease, coupled with the belief in specific etiology, opened the way for science to be brought to bear on the problems of medicine with the resultant spectacular success of which we are the beneficiaries.

Thus, in a brief period, disease classification, diagnostic methodologies, and the search for specific etiologies entered into medicine, turning it on its head. Stanley Reiser details these developments in his book, *Medicine and the Reign of Technology* (1978). Taken together, Faber's *Nosology* and Reiser's book provide an excellent means for understanding the recent past of medical history and provide a basis for predicting what the next major trends will be.

During the nineteenth and early twentieth centuries the challenge was diagnosis. Treatment was decidedly secondary. Dr. Laín Entralgo, in his book *Doctor and Patient* (1969), tells a story of the great clinician Skoda making rounds. Skoda held forth at the bedside of a patient, displaying his usual diagnostic brilliance. When one of the assistants asked him what should be done for the patient, Skoda brushed the question aside as of no importance! He, like other great physicians of those decades, felt that science had been the salvation of the profession. A new discipline (for Skoda, anatomical pathology was the base of medical knowledge) had entered medicine that saved it from the sloppy, unfounded, and uncontrolled therapeutics of purges, poultices, and phlebotomy. That was what treatment was, and that is why treatment was of no interest. Thus, science added an equally valid cognitive discipline to the moral discipline of responsibility to the patient and to the profession that had been handed down through millenia. Medicine, like the remainder of humankind, had entered the era of science and technology.

During the last forty or fifty years medicine has again been turned inside out by the rapidly expanding innovation with which we are all familiar. The fact that change is still going on hardly requires comment except to point out that one of the most recent major advances is the large-scale controlled therapeutic trial, the widespread acceptance of which is little more than a decade old.

CURRENT PROBLEMS

The effectiveness that blesses our hands would not have been possible were it not for disease classification introduced in the early nineteenth century. But a circularity is built into the system that prevents us from seeing its inadequacies. The disease classification is based on pathology—alterations in structure. Even though disease definitions that are primarily biochemical or physiological have recently become acceptable, the basic thinking is still oriented around the structural alterations of disease. Consequently, the therapeutic effectiveness of which we are justly proud is also oriented toward diseases. It should be no surprise that our care of the sick is out of balance. If some aspect of an illness is not included in the definition of the associated disease, treatment will not usually be directed at that feature of the illness. The concentration on disease and technology has contributed to a lack of understanding of the more personal and human aspects of sickness. Growing awareness of that lack and widespread desire to find a remedy are part of the reason behind the Conference on Changing Values in Medicine and this volume. However, the search for a more balanced medicine is by no means new. There is a certain irony in the fact that Rudolf Virchow, who provided the strongest evidence for the structural basis of disease, and in so doing helped bury humanism in medicine for a hundred years, was himself a committed humanist. In 1848 he wrote, "Our task is an educational one, we must train men capable of fighting the battles of humanism" (*Medicinische Reform 1848*, p. 274). In this century, the deficiencies of an orientation to disease alone have become increasingly obvious. The March 19, 1927, issue of the *Journal of the American Medical Association* carried the now famous paper by Francis Peabody, "The Care of the Patient," which states the problem posed by concentrating on disease as clearly as it has ever been written.

Over the past two generations, certainly since the 1950s, medical educators have attempted to shift the orientation of medical education and medical practice away from an almost exclusive concern with disease and technology and toward a greater concentration on patients themselves. The phrase "treat the patient as a person" has been around for so long that it has become a cliché. Note that although the phrase "a coin lesion of the lung is carcinoma until proven otherwise" has also been around for a long time, we do not call it a cliché, but rather a dictum. The difference between the two statements is that the one about the coin lesion not only provides a direction for action, but it rests on a substantial base of knowledge and recorded experience. In addition, the language of description for the lung and its lesion is by now held in common by physicians over the entire world. By contrast, "treat the patient as a person" is an imperative that rests on the common humanity of physicians and patients; it is largely unspoken, uses no universally agreed upon "professional" language, and provides no unambiguous basis for action. (Indeed, the phrase itself is somewhat ambivalent since it literally means that a patient should be treated as if a patient were a person; as in "when treating women with cancer of the breast, one should remember that they are also persons.")

It is not surprising, therefore, that these attempts to reorient the direction of the profession have not been very successful. In fact, there are even some who feel that the problem has actually worsened. These commentators point out that in recent decades medicine seems to have become increasingly technological and scientistic, and consequently more impersonal. According to that view, we take into our medical schools the most compassionate, concerned, and bright young people and turn them into "autotechnicons." While that may be a somewhat harsh viewpoint, it is certainly true that it is difficult to compete in the students' list of priorities with biochemistry or learning to do technical procedures or to read CAT scans.

During the same period that our disquiet with medicine has been growing, the world around has been in upheaval. The last two decades have seen our culture's view of science change from the source of salvation to the source of difficulties. Skepticism has replaced the former sense of trust. Paradoxically, a distinct antitechnological drift co-exists with a continued love of new products and the increased distrust of physicians noted earlier. It is startling these days to find that patients who have been seriously ill with infections often attribute their postillness fatigue to the antibiotics that cured them, instead of the illness. The drug has become the enemy, not the disease. While that may be a natural attribute of an extraordinarily healthy society, it is also an indicator of the cultural milieu.

There have also been marked changes in the traditional attitudes of Americans to their government and to authority in general (including physicians), and even in the concept of the individual, so vital to American political history. The word *individual* (the Constitution of the United States speaks of persons in the same sense), which once meant primarily someone who is equal before the law, has increasingly come to mean someone who is his or her own person— "me, myself, and I." Sameness is no longer the salient characteristic; instead, differences are the crucial feature of the concept of the individual. This is not the place to explore the profound conflicts that are introduced into American political life as a result of the change in the cultural meaning of the word *individual*. It is apposite, however, that this volume addresses an exactly parallel problem in medicine and in medical science. The social medicine movement of the 1930s addressed itself to the problem of providing all sick persons with equal care regardless of race, ethnicity, or socioeconomic status, and those are still important concerns. But now, in addition, the patient is seen to be unique and it is because of its contribution to that sick person's illness and treatment, and its relevance to that person's life, that the idiosyncratic mix of features that we know as *person* has come to demand attention. This is clumsy to write because there is no synonym for *person*; the meaning resides in the word, and the meaning has changed in the last twenty years. All those intertwined changes—technological, cultural, and political—have created the setting in which the Conference on Changing Values in Medicine took place.

FOCUS OF THE CONFERENCE

Although this conference is certainly not the first time these issues have been addressed, it does represent a fundamental change in approach to the problem of attending to persons in the medical setting. That approach is based on several beliefs. We do not think that doctors turn away from the personal within their patients because doctors do not care, or that students opt for technical means because they lose their concern and compassion. Both students and doctors act the way they do because their knowledge and skills, all hard-earned, are primarily disease oriented. When they do not attend to the personal aspects of illness and patient care, it is simply because they do not know how. They do not have the knowledge or the skills because they were not taught. In fact, beyond providing role models and the moral imperative to treat the person, faculties of medicine do not know how to teach the special skills required by the change of medicine's focus toward the sick person.

The conference and this volume are more than a restatement of the need for a medicine concerned primarily with the sick person, and they go beyond simply another cry for more humanism in medicine. Rather, these papers are based on the belief that gaps in knowledge and understanding (technical problems in one sense of that word), and not a lack of humane impulse, are what stand in the way of progress. Further, the papers reflect the conviction that these difficulties will give way before the sustained application of intellect and concern, just as have the afflictions of the sick in previous times. That our knowledge is inadequate, that the path is obscure, merely joins us to all of the history of medicine. To redress these deficiencies, to acquire the necessary knowledge and skills, individuals must make this intellectual area their primary academic concern. And for that to happen, new sources of support must be made available and medical schools must honor the endeavor. With appropriate effort we believe that these changes can and will take place. It is our hope that this volume will point to some of the many areas of research that are necessary.

PATHS TO THE FUTURE

Even if we could agree about the problems of today's medicine, we would still be a long way from being able to propose solutions. Lack of agreement about the main difficulties in modern medicine has not stemmed the tide of proposed solutions. Holistic medicine is an example of a prescription for better medical practice that has taken hold as a small social movement. The proponents of holistic medicine, however, like most critics of current medical practice, are much clearer about what they do not want medical practice to be than about what physicians should do in the future.

What are the major barriers to understanding the future of medicine in a time of change? Of the many issues identified by the authors in this volume, we believe that three stand out. First, there is the change in the status of the individual noted above. This expresses itself in medicine as a tension between two different ways of viewing the patient. In one, roles and relationships assume primary importance: the patient is regarded as someone who relates to others, the disease, the environment, the physicians, and who cannot be seen or treated apart from those relationships. In the more recent view, the patient is considered primarily as an autonomous possessor of immutable rights that override every other consideration.

The second barrier to understanding the future of medicine arises from the science that has been fundamental to the development of modern medicine. In science the objective is to understand the individual occurrence by means of a general law. But in medical practice, knowledge of what is generally the case does not tell the physician how to treat this particular patient. The problem of how to proceed from the prototypic case to the individual instance remains to be solved in a systematic manner.

The third, and perhaps most important, source of difficulty is that many of medicine's basic concepts are assumed to be so widely shared and understood that definition and analysis are unnecessary. The strength of Otto Guttentag's essay—indeed, of his life's work—is his realization that we stumble not because of failures to understand the complex, but because we fail to stop and analyze the obvious and the simple. Professor Guttentag forces us to attend to the rarely articulated but fundamental question, "Who and what is medicine all about?"

Speaking from the perspective of the attending physician—the patient's doctor—Guttentag reexamines the most basic issues of all of medicine: what is a patient, what is care, what is sickness. Step by step, he looks at every concept in the central medical equation. His paper is a distillation of the work of decades: each of its major themes—the central role of the attending physician, the physician-patient encounter, and the single disease concept or clinical entity—has been the subject of previous papers. His complex essay can most profitably be approached through the references provided at the end of his paper.

The rapid and profound transformation of medicine by scientific and technological advances over the past fifty or so years seems to have changed the role of the physician, to have made romantic but obsolete the notion of a single doctor taking care of a single patient. In assessing these developments, Walsh McDermott contends that far from diminishing the centrality of the patient's own physician, the new technology has actually thrust the doctor into an even more pivotal role. Because the use of technology begins at the bedside, a return to the centrality of the attending physician is no more romantic idyll, but is increasingly essential in order to control the use and cost of technology. Hence McDermott calls for the development of a more "discriminating medicine," with the personal physician as the key to its success.

Pedro Laín Entralgo, writing about the meaning of the word *good* in *good patient*, and James Childress in his commentary, bring us directly to the center of another of the issues critical to understanding the future of medicine. For Professor Laín Entralgo the good patient is not only a person altered by sickness, but someone who has religious, moral, and social duties which are a necessary part of the equally necessary will to get well. These duties, and the obligation to try to get well, entail certain attitudes towards the physician, the patient's own self, and the surrounding society. In the totality of these duties, obligations, and attitudes, one finds the good patient. Written with Laín Entralgo's characteristic richness and penetrating insight into patients, doctors, and medicine, his essay places more emphasis on the duties of the patient than on his or her rights. This picture is not changed by his closing insistence that to be a good patient requires a good physician.

James Childress counters these views with arguments that—although seldom so well expressed—are becoming increasingly familiar to American physicians. Professor Childress takes Laín Entralgo to task for overemphasizing the patient's duties as a patient and undervaluing the individual's rights and freedoms that, he believes, are in no way diminished by the fact of patienthood. Childress vigorously argues the position sometimes called "radical autonomy": nothing must diminish patients' rights to make autonomous choices. To speak about the will to be cured represents a kind of moral paternalism in which the value of health is seen to have priority over other goals, such as freedom. Even the use of the term *good patient*, he suggests, introduces an unnecessarily moral tone to the argument, and he offers as a substitute *responsible patient*. Although more articulate than most, Childress's plea has found many voices of late, even among physicians. This argument also has adherents in nursing.

This issue resonates in the other papers in the volume. In the discussions by Mark Siegler, Eric Cassell, and Otto Guttentag, as in the conversations of virtually all physicians, no matter what their stated position on patient autonomy, some necessary relationship between patient and doctor is presumed. Even Edmund Pellegrino, who is a forceful advocate of patient autonomy, points out that both the illness and the relationship with the physician alter the almost absolute primacy of autonomy that seems to be pictured by Childress. Pellegrino, however, resists Alasdair MacIntyre's characterization of the problem. With his usual elegant clarity, MacIntyre goes to the heart of the matter and contends that the person pictured in the radical autonomy view is, simply stated, a myth. No person exists apart from all of his or her roles or the social setting and matrix in which they are found. Autonomy, for MacIntyre, "is not ... a property of every rational agent. It is an achievement and a social achievement, as is rationality itself" (p. 95). It follows that the actions of physicians and the image of medicine they value and project will have a profound effect on the patient's ability to achieve and maintain autonomy. Does the depersonalizing bureaucracy of doctoring, organized in the name of efficiency or cost control, further enmesh patients or set them free? Will doctors be owners of the power of magic or sharers of knowledge? Is the patient an object of scientific attention or a sick person to be cared for? Alasdair MacIntyre explores all these questions and their implications in rewarding detail.

MacIntyre's paper, and indeed many of the other papers, makes it clear that certain kinds of knowledge and information which seem essential to medical practice are far from the scientific generalizations about the body and disease usually considered medical knowledge. Mark Siegler convincingly argues that clinical medicine, in contrast to research medicine, cannot be understood solely in terms of its body of scientific knowledge. He makes his point by showing that the nature and limits of clinical medicine are defined by what is essentially a personal encounter between doctor and patient. The evolution of the encounter is traced from its beginnings in the patient's decision that something is a "medical" problem to a developed relationship between doctor and patient. Dr. Siegler divides the encounter, for the purposes of analysis, into four clinical moments: the person in the prepatient phase, the initial encounter with the physician, the achievement of a negotiated accommodation between the two, and finally, the development of the doctor-patient relationship. The suggestion is advanced that the aggregation of many negotiations at the individual doctor-patient level might reveal the socially and politically acceptable norms and limits of clinical medicine. Siegler shows how political, economic, and social forces, apart from the biology of disease, determine what issues will be considered medical, but also how much latitude there is for individual negotiations between doctor and patient. MacIntyre's essay is also apposite here: he shows how the so-called nonmedical actions and attitudes of physicians bear on the care of patients. Thus, the knowledge of how those actions and attitudes work their effects, and how they can be manipulated to best advantage in the care of the sick, is legitimate medical knowledge in clinical medicine.

While it may seem odd to some to consider information about the bureaucratic setting of medical care, for example, as specifically medical knowledge, it is Kenneth Schaffner, in his commentary on Siegler, who brings us to the truly central problem with current medical knowledge. Much of the history of medical science (in common with Western thought since the Greeks) has been preoccupied with the search for universal truths. That pursuit has been, as we are all aware, spectacularly rewarding. Schaffner points out that, particularly in the domain of sick persons, there are two features of central importance with which science can deal only inadequately: individual differences and differing levels of organization (subcellular, cellular, organ, organism, roles, social system and so forth). This defect of science is crucial because no understanding of the illness of a particular patient can be achieved without reference to levels as far apart as enzyme systems and interpersonal relationships. Further, and most important as Professor Schaffner makes clear, individual differences exist and produce effects at each level. Here, stated in another manner and based on evidence from the laboratory, is one of the difficulties that faces all who try to define the good physician. Judgment is the property of applying knowledge of the universal rule to the individual instance. *Individuum est ineffabile*, the individual is unknowable. Is that an unalterable truth, or might we not try to get a little closer to a way of knowing about individuals? The problems exposed by Professor Schaffner seem stubborn, but because they are barriers to medical progress, they invite attack.

Eric Cassell suggests that at least one obstacle to knowledge about the individual patient is the physician's apparent distaste for subjective information. Further, he is concerned that medical education, and consequently medical practice, has drifted away from direct relevance to the larger dimensions of its job because "the subjective aspects of illness—what patients say, desire, think, fear, feel, and care about, and how and why they behave the way they do toward disease, doctors, symptoms, their bodies, themselves, and others—seem to be an impediment to staying at the bedside and to understanding sickness" (p. 151). After peeling away layers of this loaded issue, Cassell comes to personal meanings (the significance and importance of things to an individual, the beliefs and values attached to them) as the sense of the subjective that is at once both vital and troubling to medicine. Cassell attempts to show how personal meanings are important both diagnostically and therapeutically. After discussing aspects of the physician's subjectivity, he suggests that the personal meanings of patients can be known in all their individuality only through attentive understanding of the patient's conversation—a kind of listening very different from that in ordinary conversation and for which special training should be provided.

In commenting on Cassell, Ernan McMullin clarifies the distinctions between objective and subjective knowledge. In so doing he suggests that many of the difficulties physicians have in this area are a professional prejudice coming from the vain attempt to model medical science after physics or mathematics. Professor McMullin also questions whether there can be the systematic knowledge of the particular or individual case. He is doubtful of the possibility but suggests that the issue of a means to a reliable knowledge of the particular, like other problems raised by clinical medicine, will certainly draw increasing attention from philosophers.

The previous discussions have indicated that physicians' abilities to know about their patients and to have a more comprehensive understanding of human sickness are restricted by narrow views of what constitutes medical knowledge, as well as archaic prejudices in regard to subjective or objective ways of knowing. Stephen Toulmin, in his essay on causation, and H. Tristram Engelhardt, Jr.'s comment on Toulmin highlight another of the conceptual straitjackets that inhibit greater concern with the sick person and maintain the exclusive focus on the disease. They show that what now holds us back was previously—and not too long ago—a liberating concept. At the same time that modern disease concepts were introduced early in the nineteenth century, the concept of specific etiology was also developed. While our success with infectious diseases would seem to uphold the idea of specific etiology, Professor Toulmin shows that questions of medical causation "do not raise intellectual questions about scientific explanation as much as they do practical questions about the attribution of responsibility" (p. 65). In other words, decisions about where to intervene in the chain of events leading to sickness will follow from ideas of causation. But he further points out that from a philosophical perspective psychological, social, and political factors have no less right to attention as causes of ill health than do somatic factors. Rather, habits of thought and action, not the logic of effectiveness, maintain the concentration on physiology and bio-chemistry. These conclusions are reinforced by Engelhardt's review of the history of these issues, and his belief that by choosing where to place its accents of concern medicine creates a picture of disease that directs therapy and research. Medical accounts of causation are, thus, not value-free pictures of the world, but road maps which suggest approaches most likely to be successful for the purposes of health care.

Ideas presented by the authors in this volume suggest some of the problems that must be solved if medicine is to successfully redirect it energies towards the sick person and away from an exclusive concern with disease. It is not uncommon to end the introduction to a volume like this by suggesting that further research is necessary. It must be pointed out, however, that the kind of research that these questions require finds most physicians poorly prepared. The tools of laboratory investigation or even clinical or epidemiological study will not do. Even the habitual modes of thought of physicians will not suffice, and their prejudice against "soft" research (ultimately, something done merely with the brain) is an outright liability.

Philosophers are perhaps no better off after generations devoted largely to theoretical questions. John Ladd explores the history of the bristly relationship between medicine and philosophy in order to highlight current trends. There is no longer any doubt that there is a field of philosophy devoted to medicine and that there is a place for philosophy in medicine. It seems equally evident that Otto Guttentag no longer labors alone, as increasing numbers of physicians begin to tackle theoretical questions in clinical medicine. Professor Ladd demonstrates effectively that the contribution of philosophy to medicine (and vice versa) is by no means limited to medical ethics. Before long, one might surmise by reading his essay, the field of medical ethics which helped to create this new marriage will be but one child of the relationship. But the relationship will be strained and the reorientation of medical care primarily toward sick persons will be difficult as long as premedical and medical education remain as they are today.

Max Black's essay is a prescription for change that speaks eloquently of what can be taught to students to prepare them for a career in medicine devoted to the service of the sick. What he suggests in the way of training in communication, in teaching students methods of thought and inquiry, in grounding students in the principles of ethics and in other areas of the humanities, would seem a necessary part of premedical or medical curricula. Stanley Reiser's commentary makes the point that simply adding humanities to the curriculum of medical students, either in college or in medical school, is not sufficient; in addition, teachers must continually be able to show why technological answers alone are inadequate to provide for the care of the sick and what dilemmas will be raised by any change in the direction of medical care.

In 1896, Andrew Dickson White, who had helped Ezra Cornell found Cornell University, published a book entitled *A History of the Warfare of Science with Theology in Christendom*. In two volumes he detailed the trials overcome by science in its rise to eminence in human thought. Science and technology have enriched medicine beyond anyone's wildest expectation. But the legacy of that warfare also remains, and it has kept physicians only partially trained and patients only partially served. It is our hope that this book, by opening up questions and suggesting exciting areas for research and study, as well as showing the eminent practicality of the collaboration of medicine and philosophy, will help to restore balance to medicine and redirect physicians to their age-old calling of healing the sick.

Bibliography

Faber, K. 1923. *Nosography*. New York: Paul Hoeber.

Laín Entralgo, P. 1969. *Doctor and Patient*. New York: McGraw-Hill.

Peabody, F. 1927. "The Care of the Patient." *Journal of the American Medical Association* 88, no. 12:8 7-82.

Reiser, S. 1978. *Medicine and the Reign of Technology*. New York: Cambridge University Press.

Virchow, R. 1848. *Medizinische Reform*.

White, A.D. 1960 [1896]. *A History of the Warfare of Science with Theology in Christendom*. Mineola, NY: Dover Publications.

Part I:
The Practice of Medicine

The Nature and Limits of Clinical Medicine

Mark Siegler

This volume is dedicated to Professor Otto Guttentag, who has contributed so much to the revival of interest in the philosophy of clinical medicine. Both Professor Guttentag and I approach questions in clinical medicine from the perspective of involved participants, clinicians who are also attending physicians. But whereas Professor Guttentag describes the roles of attending physicians and the relationships between doctors and patients from what he calls a "conceptual" or ideal perspective, I will examine these issues in more concrete and practical terms.[1] My point of departure is a passage from one of Professor Guttentag's recent papers: "What then is the irreducible given in 'health care'? The answer may be formulated as follows: It is the positive, active response by someone who is convinced of being able to respond effectively to another's overt or hidden request: 'Help me in the care of my health.' However else the situation may be defined, someone calls to have health needs fulfilled, and someone responds to this call" (1978).

THEORIES OF HEALTH AND DISEASE

Physicians and philosophers have developed many theories of health and disease. Such constructions attempt to describe the nature of health and disease, and the descriptions are often used to prescribe the proper range and scope of clinical medicine. These analyses often turn on the issue of whether disease is an objective biological state, describable and verifiable by objective criteria, or, alternatively, whether disease is relative to social and cultural values.

For example, in defending the "traditional" medical model, Seldin (1977) has argued that modern medicine ought to restrict its scope to those medical, surgical, and psychiatric conditions for which effective drug or surgical therapy is available. Medicine, he claims, should be narrowly disease oriented, and should not take on a variety of social or political missions which it is not capable of accomplishing. According to this view, the goal of medicine is in the maintenance or restoration of health. Leon Kass (1975, p. 13) has suggested that the goal of medicine, or at least the "end" of the physician's art, is "health—or if you prefer, the healthy human being...." Kass dismisses other goals, such as happiness, behavior modification, and death prevention, as inappropriate and extraneous to the central mission of medicine.

In contrast to these positions describing limited goals for medicine, others contend that medicine has been far too narrow in scope and that a broader model is needed, one which George Engel (1977) has called a "biopsychosocial" model of medicine. According to Engel, "The psychosocial unity of man requires that the physician accept the responsibility to evaluate whatever problems the patient presents and recommend a course of action including referrals to other helping professions. Hence the physician's basic professional knowledge and skill must span the social, psychological and biological, for his decisions and actions on the patient's behalf involve all three" (p. 133).

H. Tristram Engelhardt, Jr. takes an equally broad view, claiming that the historical tradition of medicine has encouraged physicians to respond to the full range of patient complaints: "One must, in fact, somewhat circularly say that the world of medicine is defined by the medical complaints of people and medical complaints are what medicine could in principle address ... The art of medicine is the art of practicing a skill in a way that effectively treats the complaints of patients" (1979, p. 227). For both Engel and Engelhardt, the role of medicine is to provide effective help to individuals who "present" to the medical system with self-defined medical problems.

I do not wish to deny the importance of developing conceptual models to account for actual behavior or the potential usefulness of such models in modifying behavior in the future. If agreed upon, the models could influence the medical profession's own sense of the range and extent of its medical obligations. A professional consensus about the limits of medicine might eventually be reflected in medical education—beginning with the process of selecting medical students and including their undergraduate and postgraduate education—as well as in the medical marketplace. Further, if health planners and legislators could agree on a particular theoretical model (whether or not the profession concurred entirely), practical limits could be established, primarily through financial mechanisms, on the scope of clinical medical activities.

My concern is that these theoretical accounts of the nature and limits of clinical medicine never quite come to grips with the actualities of medical practice. I will therefore pursue a different program, beginning not with theories of health and disease, but rather with my perception of how clinical medicine works in the realities of daily practice. Before any theory of physicians' actions can be formulated, it is essential to understand how physicians currently function and how they describe and justify their actions.

Before proceeding, it is important to point out the distinction between a "health problem" and "a problem in clinical medicine."[2] My own view is that the legitimate goal of clinical medicine is the pursuit of both physical and mental health. However, clinical medicine is merely one means by which health can be preserved or regained. In the absence of clinical intervention health can be maintained or regained by improving living conditions, nutrition, sanitation, or education, and by strengthening an individual's personal responsibility for the maintenance of his own health. In short, not all health problems are appropriate problems of or for clinical medicine. (Some health problems would be legitimate problems of clinical medicine if they ever came to the attention of the traditional medical system. However, because of the inaccessibility of health services, or an individual's failure to recognize problems as medical, or his decision to seek treatment in nonmedical systems, these problems may never become problems for clinical medicine. Thus, a patient with asthma who is being treated by a physician has both a health problem and a clinical medical problem. By contrast, an asthmatic who goes to church to pray for the relief of symptoms may have a health problem, but does not have a clinical medical problem.)

CLINICAL MEDICINE AND THE
DOCTOR-PATIENT ACCOMMODATION

The thesis of this paper is that the nature of clinical medicine is not an entity to be discovered like a truth of nature, but that it is defined and created in the context of a doctor-patient accommodation. There is no single "nature of clinical medicine," but many such natures. What counts as a problem of clinical medicine is mutually decided upon in a doctor-patient accommodation which may lead to a deeper, longer lasting doctor-patient relationship. Without such a relationship there do not exist problems in clinical medicine, even though there may exist health problems, diseases, or even problems in preventive, social, community, or investigative medicine. Clinical medicine, then, refers to accommodations between individual physicians and patients which are designed to achieve mutually agreed upon goals.

The determination that a problem falls within the boundaries of clinical medicine (rather than that it is a disease or a health problem) is an elaborate process and is usually the result of a mutually agreed upon transaction between patient and physician. While the physician's eventual agreement with the patient that a problem is a medical problem usually decides the case, many preliminary developments must precede that determination. In general, a problem becomes one for clinical medicine only when the doctor and patient agree that it is one. If either the patient or the physician claims that a medical problem does not exist, then, with rare exceptions,[3] for their purposes the issue is not a problem of clinical medicine. While I recognize that these determinations are constrained by political, economic, and social forces, there nevertheless remains enormous latitude for negotiations between the individual patient and physician.

These negotiations, carried on by thousands of physicians who interact with millions of patients, determine the nature and limits of clinical medicine at the level of the individual doctor and patient. In addition, by aggregation, they set the societally accepted norms of the nature and limits of clinical medicine. Are there no universally accepted standards about which problems are appropriate for clinical medicine? I suggest that in this period of social uncertainty and change, which has already witnessed remarkable changes in medicine and in the traditional model of the doctor-patient relationship, both the public and physicians may lack a clear and uniform consensus on what constitutes the proper nature and limits of clinical medicine. In this context, a degree of uncertainty will prevail and neither patient nor physician may be able to appeal to fixed standards in deciding whether it is appropriate to enter into a doctor-patient accommodation.

In contemporary American society, many of the final decisions about medical care remain in the control of patients and doctors. We will examine the nature and limits of clinical medicine in this context by analyzing a routine encounter between a patient and a doctor: the occasion on which an individual "presents" to a physician with a self-defined medical problem. This analysis applies to typical encounters in the office, clinic, or hospital, but would, of course, require modification to account for acute or emergency situations.

THE FOUR CLINICAL MOMENTS IN THE
DOCTOR-PATIENT ENCOUNTER

To explore the thesis that a problem is one of clinical medicine only when the patient and the doctor agree that it is one, I will divide the medical encounter into four conceptual moments or stages: (1) the person in a prepatient phase; (2) the physician in the context of his initial encounter with the person who now presents as a patient; (3) the doctor-patient accommodation; and (4) the doctor-patient relationship. These are conceptual rather than chronological moments because they attempt to distinguish, for purposes of analysis, elements of an interconnected process that begins when patient and physician first meet, or in fact, when they first communicate. Nevertheless, most of the prepatient phase of this encounter is chronologically prior to the physician's involvement; there is also considerable action in the second clinical moment, the physician phase, which is required before a physician-patient accommodation can be concluded. In this paper I will concentrate primarily on the prepatient phase (the first clinical moment), and on the doctor-patient accommodation (the third clinical moment). I will comment only briefly on the doctor-patient relationship, primarily to distinguish this final clinical moment from the doctor-patient accommodation.

The First Clinical Moment: The Prepatient Phase of Clinical Medicine

The prepatient phase of clinical medicine represents the first clinical moment. The determination by an individual that he has a health problem must precede the actual medical encounter; thus, it represents a necessary, although not a sufficient, step in the decision that the problem is appropriate to clinical medicine. The perception that one is ill and the decision to seek medical help are influenced by social, cultural, political, and economic factors, in addition to the biological manifestations of the perceived state of ill health (Parsons 1951; Merton 1957).

The prepatient phase almost always includes attention to certain bodily sensations, that is, symptoms, the persistence of symptoms, and the effect such symptoms have on disrupting the ordinary activities of the individual and the social group. In addition, before deciding that a particular sensation or feeling is one that should be attended to by physicians rather than, for example, by priests or teachers or social workers, individuals will have considered their own values and beliefs and those of their immediate family and community, as well as the availability, cost, and quality of medical care. To understand the self-definition of illness by the prospective patient, it is instructive to examine Tolstoi's short novel, *The Death of Ivan Il'ich*. In the early chapters of this work Tolstoi permits the reader to observe the unfolding of the first clinical moment, the process by which Ivan Il'ich becomes a patient.

Tolstoi's novel recounts the life, and particularly the death, of a civil servant, a judge in imperial Russia, Ivan Il'ich. In chapter 3 of that novel, Ivan Il'ich has been passed over for a promotion and is now almost in despair: "Ivan Il'ich, for the first time in his life, expressed not merely ennui, but an unendurable depression, and arrived at the conclusion that to live like this was impossible, and that it was indispensable for him to adopt some decisive measure at once"

(p. 184). At this stage Ivan Il'ich did not decide to seeek medical care for his new sensations of profound depression. Instead, "After passing a sleepless night ... he resolved to go to St. Petersburg, and try to get transferred into another ministry, in order to punish those persons who did not appreciate him" (p. 184). Ivan Il'ich thus defined his problem as a social problem, or in the case of one working for government, as a political problem, but he clearly did not consider that he was suffering a medical illness of depression or that he should visit a physician with his problem. Once he assigned the problem to a particular category, that is, as a social or political matter, he immediately sought to resolve it in this context.

Later in chapter 3, Ivan Il'ich unexpectedly received a spectacular promotion and was delightedly furnishing his new home. While climbing on a ladder to arrange some curtains, he stumbled and knocked his side against the handle of a window frame. "The bruise hurt him a little, but the pain soon passed off. All this time, indeed, Ivan Il'ich felt particularly bright and well. He wrote his wife: 'I feel that fifteen of my years have leaped from off my shoulders' " (pp. 188-89). Even though Ivan Il'ich had received a definite physical injury—a bruise which caused pain—again he did not seek medical attention. Perhaps it was his happiness over his promotion that allowed him to state, despite his new and painful injury, that he felt fifteen years younger.

Some weeks after the injury to his side, Ivan Il'ich's wife, newly returned from a stay in the country, inquired how he had come to fall, and he laughingly explained: "I have not been a gymnast for nothing, anyone else would have been killed, and I merely struck myself here; if you touch it, it pains, but it is passing away already, it is a simple bruise" (pp. 189-90). Thus, even after discussing the injury in a social setting with his wife, Ivan Il'ich did not perceive himself as ill; nor, for that matter, did his wife, and she concurred implicitly with his decision not to seek medical attention.

Here is the situation in chapter 4:

> They were all well. Ivan Il'ich sometimes said indeed that he had a bad taste in his mouth, and something was not quite right, but one could hardly call that illness. But this little indisposition happened to increase, and passed, not yet into downright illness, but into a feeling of constant aching in the side, accompanied by lowness of spirits. This lowness of spirits kept on increasing and increasing, and began to destroy that easy, pleasant, and decorous manner of life which had become an institution in the family of the Golivins (pp. 194-95).

Even with a bad taste in his mouth, persistent and worsening pain in his side, and a general depression and lassitude—in fact, later in the chapter we learn that he also had experienced a loss of appetite and a severe irascibility that troubled his whole family and even threatened the stability of his unhappy but stable marriage—despite all this, he never arrived at a self-determination that he was ill. Why was that so? I am not convinced that his failure to self-define an illness was a result of psychological fear or denial. Nor do I think a prevailing vision of health and disease was responsible. Rather, it simply never occurred to Ivan Il'ich that he was really ill, or as Tolstoi puts it, "downright ill."

It is fascinating to discover how and why Ivan Il'ich finally decided to see a doctor. He and his wife had been having terrible scenes, usually at dinner, when he complained of the food and did not eat. After one of these scenes, he felt that he had been unjust to his wife and apologized, saying that he was irritable "because he did not feel well. She said to him that if he were ill he ought to be cured, and insisted that he should go see a famous doctor. He went" (p. 196).

Ultimately the decision to seek medical counsel was reached because Ivan Il'ich had a sense of not feeling well and because his wife urged him to seek medical attention and cure. But Ivan Il'ich and his wife were not identifying the pain, or bad taste, or loss of appetite as the illness; instead they were focusing on his irritability and ill temper and the impact of these on the family's tranquility. It appears that Ivan Il'ich sought medical attention because of the influence of his family—his wife's urging—and perhaps because entering the medical system offered a potentially extenuating excuse for his aberrant behavior. He had obviously sensed that something was not right physically, but it required a direct challenge from his wife to force him to act on his perception.

Tolstoi's *Ivan Il'ich* provides us with an insightful picture of the prepatient phase of an unfolding illness. It suggests the complex interplay between the biological complaints of pain in the side, loss of appetite, a bad taste in the mouth; the psychological concomitants of these physical pains, that is, bad temper and irascibility; and the social and family dislocation that cumulatively led to a decision— urged on him by his wife within the family context—to seek medical attention. More generally, this description of the early phases of Ivan Il'ich's illness and his decision to seek medical help suggests the following generalizations concerning the prepatient phase or first clinical moment:

1. The distinction between a problem of health and a nonhealth matter is frequently obscure.
2. Social, cultural, and psychological factors can strongly influence an individual's judgment that he has a health problem rather than a problem whose relief should be sought from other agencies, or indeed, that he has any problem at all.
3. Even if a problem is actually perceived as a health problem, one

may choose not to make it a problem of clinical medicine by not presenting it to physicians. Individuals can define a problem as a nonmedical one even when severe disease exists.

4. Different individuals can define similar conditions in different ways, just as one individual can, at different times, define the same condition in different ways.

This brings us to the second clinical moment, when the physician first enters the picture and must begin to respond to the person who presents as a patient with a problem that has been self-defined as a medical one.

The Second Clinical Moment: Data Gathering and Data Reduction

Of the initial encounter between patient and physician, David Mechanic has written, "People visit the physician because they have a problem; most frequently they come because they believe they are ill. In one sense, at least, all persons seeking advice from a physician and presenting a symptom are 'diseased.' There is something in their life condition that impels them to seek help" (1978, p. 418).

From a patient's perspective, the issue appears settled at the time he requests help: his problem should be counted and responded to as a medical problem. Nevertheless, I believe that in these circumstances the physician's response is guarded and reserved. In many instances the physician is suspicious of the patient and may question (at least in his own mind) why the patient has chosen to appear at this time and whether the patient has a clinical medical problem. While some might regard this suspicion as contrary to the medical duty to respond to a patient's request to "Help me in the care of my health ..." (Guttentag 1978), or even as an inappropriate extension of the physician's expertise (Veatch 1973), that view is misguided. This questioning stage of the physician's thinking represents a crucial technical step. The physician must determine precisely why the patient chose to present at this time, as well as the nature of the patient's symptom formation. Psychiatrists are quite adept at these analyses, particularly for psychological symptoms, but other clinicians pursue the same conceptual analysis for physical as well as psychological problems.[4]

We have already indicated that the patient's determination that a problem is medical is based on the interaction of biological, psychological, and cultural factors. Now the physician must embark on the difficult task of disentangling the factors that led to this visit, in order to determine for himself whether the patient has found his way to the proper institutional setting—that is, a medical setting— and whether the patient's problem is a "medical" one.

An essential part of this process is to determine the iatrotropic stimulus, the immediate event or events that convinced the patient to seek medical attention at this time (Feinstein 1967, p. 141-55). For example, in the case of Ivan Il'ich, the iatrotropic stimulus was family disharmony and, incidentally, an ache in his side and a strange taste in his mouth.

Simultaneously, the physician often attempts to make another and even more problematic judgment: whether this patient will be a "good patient," one who is able to work with the physician in a mutually satisfactory way, or a "problem patient." Many would prefer to ignore these emotionally charged issues, but I am convinced that such evaluative judgments occur routinely when physicians meet new patients (Cassell 1975).

What usually follows after the patient's initial presentation is a process that we have come to call the clinical method, a process whose efficacy has been established since the Hippocratic era. The two central components of the clinical method are data gathering, and data reduction and diagnosis. Although the clinical method may appear to some to be a mechanical procedure, both of its components, but especially the data-gathering phase, require a considerable amount of personal interaction and an exchange of information about technical as well as value-laden concerns between the seeker of medical care— the patient—and the individual who assumes the responsibility to provide such care—the physician.

Data gathering. The heart of data gathering occurs in the verbal and paraverbal exchanges between the patient and physician. Expert clinicians agree that no laboratory tests or technological innovations in medicine can compare to the efficiency and effectiveness of a skilled clinician's history and physical examination as tools for gathering information about patients' problems. Medical students learn very early that most diagnoses, perhaps 70 to 90 percent, are made on the basis of the medical history. This stage of the clinical encounter is absolutely and critically dependent on the interaction of two persons. By contrast, a patient-computer encounter or the collection of a written medical history questionnaire is an inadequate substitute for the interaction of the patient with a sensitive and skilled physician.[5]

The success of the data-gathering phase of the second clinical moment depends upon the interaction of the patient and doctor and on their ability to communicate effectively. As Tumulty (1970) suggests, the measure of a clinician's skill is his ability to communicate successfully with a broad and diverse group of patients. It is essential to acknowledge and to appreciate that individual responses—some conscious and some subconscious—of patients to physicians and physicians to patients can modify the effectiveness of the doctor-patient interaction.

Data reduction and diagnosis. The second stage of the clinical method is designed to reduce the enormous amount of information obtained from the history, physical examination, and laboratory studies to a useful and workable amount. The data are structured and classified according to standard taxonomies as the clinician engages in the process of differential diagnosis in order to identify as a disease the complaint with which the patient has presented. Even while attempting to generate a diagnosis, the physician is simultaneously testing the complaints to determine whether the patient legitimately falls within the clinical medical model. The second moment is not an end in itself but is a necessary preliminary step in deciding whether to proceed to the succeeding clinical moments: the doctor-patient accommodation and the doctor-patient relationship.

The second clinical moment, the patient's encounter with the physician, has traditionally been regarded as the doctor's "turf" and is too often characterized as "cold," "analytic," "objective," "rational," "reductionistic," and "scientific." But even while the physician may act as an objective scientist, an enormous amount of human and personal interaction is occurring between patient and doctor. The task of eliciting a medical history is no job for machines, for it requires the profound subtlety that only trained, sensitive humans can bring to it. As Pedro Laín Entralgo (1969) has indicated in his analysis of the doctor-patient relationship, the relationship commences when patient and physician look at each other and interact for the first time, and it deepens during the physical examination phase.

Nor do I believe that the data reduction phase, which generates a diagnosis and a differential diagnosis, is a mechanical process that can be delegated to a well-functioning and adequately programmed computer. Kenneth Schaffner has pointed out that in reaching taxonomic designations of disease, "Individuality is filtered out, usually employing a statistical methodology. What is left are important multi-level generalizations, absolutely necessary for medical science, that then have to be reindividualized by the physician.... [It] is the disease which is individualized in the patient which constitutes the illness which the physician must treat" (1979, p. 8). Although clinical medicine may utilize theories in this clinical stage, it is not wedded to theories, but to caring for patients. Thus, even the apparently scientific and mechanical second clinical moment—like the first clinical moment—is full of personal drama, and it leads inexorably to the individualization of the patient that is the central event in the third clinical phase, the doctor-patient accommodation.

The Third Clinical Moment: The Doctor-Patient Accommodation.

The third clinical moment encompasses the negotiations that may culminate in a doctor-patient accommodation. My thesis is that the nature of clinical medicine is defined and created in the context of this accommodation, which must be mutually agreed upon by both participants. Medicine is not defined solely by its scientific knowledge base or its technological capabilities. There is a close parallel between my definition of clinical medicine and Professor Guttentag's claim "that medicine deals with the care of health of human beings by human beings" (1985, p. 110). For it is the immediate involvement of at least two human personalities that instantaneously distinguishes clinical medicine from a host of other activities in which technological skills based on scientific discoveries are ultimately applied for human benefit—activities such as bridge building, architecture, and veterinary medicine.

The participants in a doctor-patient accommodation have been prepared for their encounter by a series of preliminary experiences which have led the patient to seek counsel from the physician (the first clinical moment) and have prepared the physician to serve the patient as knowledgeable counselor. From the moment the patient originally presented to the physician (the second clinical moment), testing and evaluation have been carried out by both parties. In the stage I refer to as the doctor-patient accommodation, a joint decision is reached as to whether *this* doctor will agree to care for *this* patient, and as to whether *this* patient will place his care in the hands of *this* physician. Only if this third stage, the doctor-patient accommodation, is successfully concluded can the fourth phase, the doctor-patient relationship, be initiated.

During the negotiations that may culminate in a doctor-patient accommodation, the patient and the physician are each thinking silently about a series of questions; affirmative answers will encourage them to conclude the accommodation. The patient is asking: Are my symptoms serious (my fear) or trivial (my hope)? Is this doctor a good doctor (for me)? Can he help me? Simultaneously, the physician wants to know: Are the patient's symptoms "real"? Does the patient have a "disease" or just a "problem of living" which may not be a matter proper for medicine? Is the patient's problem serious (his fear) or trivial (his hope)? Is this patient a good patient (for me)? Can I help him and still remain loyal to my obligations as a physician and as a participant in the medical enterprise?

The patient's choice. There are many reasons why a patient might decide not to continue with a particular doctor. For example, if the doctor had a poor bedside manner, seemed incompetent, had the wrong diplomas on the wall (or none at all), maintained a shabby office, charged excessive fees, had too long a queue, or lacked the proper hospital privileges, the patient might choose to go elsewhere. At least in our current medical system, the patient has a choice. The patient selected this doctor initially, but if he becomes dissatisfied, he can vote with his feet. Though we may disagree about such empirical questions as whether our system truly provides all patients with free choices of physicians, or how frequently patients as a class exercise options to find another doctor, we would agree that the possibility for switching from one physician to another does exist.

The physician's choice. The physician's decision to enter a doctor-patient accommodation is also critical, although in many regards the physician is less free to choose than the patient. Legally, a doctor-patient accommodation probably exists from the first encounter with the patient; morally, a therapeutic relationship has begun at the moment doctor and patient first see each other, or perhaps at the moment the patient makes an appointment. Despite these restraints, it is not only appropriate, but also obligatory, for the physician to make a conscious decision that he will or will not assume the care of the person who asks for medical assistance.

The physician's decision is based, first, on an assessment of his ability to help the patient, and second, on his concept of professional standards and norms of behavior. Theories of health and disease are often a third consideration. Thus, the negotiated accommodation between doctor and patient balances the needs of patients (the physician's responsibility to individuals) and the science of medicine (the physician's responsibility to his professional standards). In this context, the "good" physician can be viewed as one who successfully balances his responsibility to individual patients with his responsibility to his art.

Medical science aims to explain physiological or biochemical derangements or to label diseases; clinical medicine, by contrast, aims to do something for patients, such as curing or caring or educating. In the development of the doctor-patient accommodation, the conscientious physician asks himself two interrelated questions: Can anything be done for this patient's problem? Can *I* do anything for this patient's problem? The first question stems from the distinction between the diagnosis of the disease and the possibilities for therapeutic intervention.[6] The second question transcends the issue of whether treatment is available; it focuses instead on the patient's potential to benefit from a therapeutic encounter with a particular physician. In deciding whether he will be able to help, the physician takes three important factors into account: technical competence, the quality of his personal interaction with the patient, and the mutual compatability of their therapeutic goals.

The physician begins by assessing the adequacy of his technical competence. In many cases the answer is obvious. For example, a patient with abdominal pain from acute appendicitis clearly requires the skills of a surgeon, not an internist, while a patient with abdominal pain from diabetic ketoacidosis is usually better off tended by an internist rather than a surgeon. In more subtle cases, the same principle may apply; that is, some physicians, even when trained in a specific area, do not do as well as some of their colleagues in caring for certain kinds of cases. Consider the treatment of irritable bowel syndrome, one of the most common gastrointestinal disorders. All physicians are trained to deal with this problem, and internists regularly see many of these cases. Yet some clinicians achieve remarkable success in caring for patients with this syndrome, while others are unable to deal easily or successfully with these patients. What is required is not merely competence derived from appropriate training, but competent performance. For some reason, psychiatrists seem more willing than other physicians to refer cases to colleagues whose skills are better suited to a particular patient's needs.

A second factor that can lead the physician to decide he is unable to help is the quality of his personal interaction with the patient. Just as some physicians react negatively to specific diseases or categories of diseases, so can physicians react negatively to individual patients or even categories of patients. Discrimination against categories of individuals is inexcusable and must be overcome. But the negative response to individuals is a personal response that cannot always be masked by the professional aura that envelops the meeting of the doctor and patient. Among my patients, there are some for whom I have a very deep affection, others whom I find agreeable, and those whom I frankly dislike. Although I strive to care for each of my patients to the best of my ability, there is little doubt that I am more effective as a person and as a physician with those patients I like. We resonate well together: they know how I am thinking and feeling, and I apprehend how they are doing more directly than in other cases. They know they have a friend as well as a doctor. These observations echo the eloquent passages of Dr. Laín Entralgo when he speaks of medical *phillia*, a deep medical friendship, as being at the heart of the relationship between doctor and patient (Laín Entralgo 1969).

I would suggest that a physician can justifiably decide not to enter an elective doctor-patient accommodation (in precisely the way the patient might decide) when, because of personality clashes, it will be impossible to achieve an effective working relationship. (All such considerations collapse, of course, in the face of direct patient needs.) Still, even the most difficult and "self-abusing"[7] patients will be better off when cared for by empathetic physicians who are eager to enter a doctor-patient accommodation than by physicians who are forced to deliver services (Groves 1978). The recruitment and training of such empathetic physicians is a major responsibility of the medical profession.

A third reason for deciding not to enter into a doctor-patient accommodation is the physician's discovery that the goals and ends being pursued by the patient are incompatible with his own goals in treating the patient. This incompatibility can lead the physician to conclude that he will be unable to help the patient and that it would be better not to enter an accommodation. Physicians must be sensitive to the different goals that can underlie requests for medical attention. While it may appear obvious that what patients desire is a restoration of health, a variety of alternative ends are possible, for example reduction in disability, dysfunctional states, or deformity; relief of pain or suffering; increased knowledge (such as the name of a disease or its prognosis); reassurance and calming of family members; secondary gains of money (e.g., disability insurance) or power (e.g., that derived from being dependent) or revenge. At the initial meeting all of these are potential goals, and the physician must determine which ones are important for this particular patient.

A patient may also have philosophical or religious goals that take precedence over health-related goals; for example, some patients value autonomy and self-determination more than the restoration of bodily health. Thus, for a Jehovah's Witness on the brink of death from hemorrhage, the right to pursue religious beliefs and the goal of eternal salvation may be considerably more important than being transfused and having one's life saved. When the goals of the patient and those of the physician are profoundly different and not reconcilable by good-faith negotiations, the physician may decide that he is simply not able to assist the patient in achieving the goals desired from the medical encounter. In such instances the physician is once again obligated not to enter into a doctor-patient accommodation.

This obligation to make a conscious choice is rooted in the fundamental objective of medical care. Because medicine is aimed at achieving desirable ends for patients, it is to the patient's advantage for physicians to exercise discretion and prudence in selecting persons they wish to treat. It would be counterproductive to initiate a doctor-patient accommodation if there are strong reasons to believe it will not be successful.

A physician may also decide not to enter a doctor-patient accommodation if the patient's demands conflict with the physician's view of professional responsibility or his perception of what is involved in being a "good" doctor. Physicians are not required to act illegally or immorally even if patients ask them to do so, as, for example, when physicians are asked to lie or deceive so the patient can receive benefits, or to justify unnecessary tests or hospitalization. Illegal or immoral demands are legitimate grounds for a physician to refuse to initiate or to discontinue a doctor-patient accommodation.[8,9] A more difficult situation arises when the patient's demands are neither immoral nor illegal, but challenge a physician's personal notion of what it is to be a good doctor. Consider the following case from my own experience.

A twenty-six-year-old woman in her first trimester of pregnancy experienced a worsening of her mild, nondisfiguring psoriasis. She had been receiving conventional treatment but had read that methotrexate therapy, although considerably more toxic, was more convenient to take and offered a high response rate. Methotrexate is a known teratogenic substance and is contraindicated in pregnant women. The patient was informed of this but nevertheless demanded methotrexate treatment. I refused and a doctor-patient accommodation was never achieved.

In this case, I refused to acquiesce to the patient's demand because I believed the requested methotrexate therapy was inappropriate, unnecessary, excessive, and dangerous. The risks outweighed the potential benefits. I refused, in other words, because the request conflicted with my view of what a good physician—one responsible to his patients, to himself, and to his art—would do under these circumstances.

The traits involved in being a good physician are difficult to define and even more difficult to justify, but they nevertheless exist. We would think badly, for example, of a physician who treated tension headaches with morphine, or painful, chronic rheumatoid arthritis with high doses of corticosteroids. Although in both instances the patient's symptoms would be suppressed, we would criticize the physician's poor judgment in selecting unnecessarily powerful drugs that exposed the patient to unacceptable risks. And our poor opinion would not change even if we learned that the treatment had been demanded by the patient. Knowing that the physician was persuaded by a demanding patient to act in a way that was contrary to the physician's own concept of good medicine might lead us to an even harsher indictment: that this physician lacked a "medical conscience."

Let me turn now to a third reason why a good physician might decide not to enter a doctor-patient accommodation: the conviction that the patient's problems are not medical problems and ought not be addressed by clinical medicine. This situation differs from the earlier one in which the patient and the physician desired different and incompatible ends but agreed that their encounter had found its way to the appropriate institutional setting, that is, the medical setting. A physician's decision that a particular complaint is or is not a medical problem is based upon the diagnosis he has reached, his sense of the patient's motivations for coming to the doctor, and his own beliefs and values. While some of these values may be broadly shared by society (for example, certain norms about health and disease), others may be quite particular to physicians as a group or to an individual physician.

I am not suggesting that we are dealing here with a radical relativism, for there do exist some widely shared notions of what constitute medical problems. It would not be difficult to muster a consensus that a broken leg, hemorrhagic shock, the need for open-heart surgery, acute appendicitis, and congestive heart failure are problems that fall within the purview of clinical medicine. However, we would likely discover widely divergent views about whether the following are properly medical matters: amniocentesis for gender identification, the management of exogenous obesity, drug addiction, control of hyperactive children, poverty and malnutrition, nonspecific anxiety in middle-aged persons, elective abortions, aging, accident-proneness, unhappiness, and unattractiveness. Models of health and disease, either those articulated by philosophers or those taught to physicians in medical school, probably find their widest application at this stage of the doctor-patient encounter. Whether a physician places a particular patient's complaints within or outside of the sphere of clinical medicine depends, in part, on the theoretical view to which he subscribes.

Thus, the nature and limits of clinical medicine are defined in the interaction and negotiation between patient and physician which occurs in the third clinical moment, the doctor-patient accommodation. From the patient's viewpoint, what is sought is help in the care of his health. From the physician's perspective, what is important is being able to provide help to the patient while remaining loyal to his professional responsibilities to the science and art of medicine. The greatest practitioners of clinical medicine are those who most successfully balance these competing loyalties.

The Fourth Clinical Moment: The Doctor-Patient Relationship

The achievement of a doctor-patient relationship, the fourth clinical moment, depends entirely on the satisfactory conclusion of a doctor-patient accommodation. The relationship is distinguished from the accommodation by its duration, depth, and maturity. Although there are no formal signs to acknowledge its existence, physicians and patients usually recognize that their medical relationship has advanced and entered a new phase. The progression from a doctor-patient accommodation to a doctor-patient relationship is not simply temporal, for not all accommodations eventually result in permanent doctor-patient relationships. The essential feature of a doctor-patient relationship is the exchange of a deep bond of trust between patient and doctor. The exchange may occur at any time: on the very first visit, after many years, or not at all. If and when the exchange of trust occurs, it serves to stabilize the medical relationship during periods of new and difficult stress.

Previous descriptions of the doctor-patient relationship (e.g., Szasz and Hollender 1956; Veatch 1972) tend to regard it as a stable, unchanging interactional system in which the relationship of physicians to patients is relatively fixed and static. I am proposing a much more dynamic model. In my view, the stability of the doctor-patient relationship is tested constantly by the need to achieve repeated accommodations concerning new developments that inevitably arise. Thus, the doctor-patient accommodation and the doctor-patient relationship are always in a state of dynamic equilibrium; mutual trust tends to drive the equation toward maintaining the doctor-patient relationship, but new circumstances constantly force the patient and physician to reassess the stability of their ongoing medical relationship. For example, changes in the patient (e.g., the development of new diseases, attitudes, or demands), changes in the physician (e.g., a change in specialization, restriction of practice, or the development of new attitudes), or changes in their trust of one another may result in a failure to achieve a doctor-patient accommodation of a new issue and lead to a dissolution of the previously established doctor-patient relationship. The model of medicine implied by my emphasis on the need for physicians and patients to achieve repeated accommodations is one of mutuality and voluntariness. Mutual consent is thus a necessary condition for morally acceptable medical practice and is essential in defining the nature and limits of clinical medicine.

CONCLUSION

In Book IV of *The Laws*, Plato describes two different kinds of doctor-patient relationships. The first, medical care provided to slaves, is rigid and mechanical; it lacks preliminary discussion and has no regard for the individuality of the patient. "A physician who treats slaves never gives him any account of his complaints, nor asks him for any; he gives him some empiric injunction with an air of finished knowledge in the brusque fashion of a dictator, and then is off in hot haste to the next ailing slave ..." (1934, p. 104). Plato contrasts this mechanical approach of caring for slaves with the accommodation achieved between physicians and free men: "[The physician to free men] treats their disease by going into things thoroughly from the beginning in a scientific way and takes the patient and his family into confidence. Thus he learns something from the sufferers, and at the same time instructs the invalid to the best of his powers. He does not give prescriptions until he has won the patient's support, and when he has done so, he steadily aims at producing complete restoration to health by persuading the sufferer into compliance ..." (pp. 104-05).

The best clinical medicine, Plato tells us, is practiced when these essential concerns have been discussed by patient and doctor. In this regard, the doctor-patient accommodation serves as a crucial preamble to the formation of a just and effective doctor-patient relationship. The practice of a personal and individual medicine demands loyalty and commitment between patient and doctor. It is the kind of medicine in which every patient should have a personal physician who serves as a friend, counselor, and advocate.

Changes that are now occurring in medicine appear to be leading in different directions. On the one hand, medical centers are training many more primary care physicians, enough perhaps to assure that every person will be able to have such a personal physician. On the other hand, medicine is clearly becoming more bureaucratic and political. These changes may modify the patient-centered medicine that currently exists and change the delicate doctor-patient relationship from a negotiated accommodation to an impersonal contract between clients and providers. At this juncture it is difficult to predict how and whether the changing values alluded to in the title of this volume will affect the value and nature of the doctor-patient accommodation—a personal relationship which, I have argued, currently and rightly defines the nature and limits of clinical medicine.

Notes

I wish to express my thanks to the audience at the Conference on Changing Values in Medicine for their valuable criticisms and suggestions. I am grateful to Prof. Kenneth F. Schaffner and Prof. Andrew Jameton for their constructive comments on earlier drafts. Most of all, I want to thank my friend and colleague, Eric Cassell, for his assistance and invaluable guidance. My debt to Dr. Cassell derives from personal discussions and from the superb analysis of the doctor-patient relationship in his book, *The Healer's Art*.

1. In commenting on the concrete realities of everyday practice, I am following several modern reflective clinicians, particularly Cassell (1976), Laín Entralgo (1969), Pellegrino (1979), and Guttentag (1978, 1985).

The distinction I am drawing between Guttentag's "ideal perspective" and my own "concrete and practical" perspective is to an extent artificial and is used here only as a heuristic to suggest the general directions of this paper. Reflective clinicians cannot help but describe simultaneously how their task is actually performed. For the purposes of this paper, I try to adopt a descriptive, empirical approach to the nature of clinical medicine, but may on occasion slip into normative statements about how clinical medicine should ideally function. I am not entirely apologetic for such lapses; they may reveal interesting truths.

2. See Kass's essay (1975) for an exemplary analysis of the concept of health and a discussion of some of the relationships between medical practice and the pursuit of health. Kass concludes an extended discussion about health with the following statement:

> To sum up: Health is a natural standard or norm—not a moral norm, not a "value" as opposed to a "fact," not an obligation, but a state of being that reveals itself in activity as a standard of bodily excellence or fitness, relative to each species and to some extent to individuals, recognizable if not definable, and to some extent attainable. If you prefer a more simple formulation, I would say that health is "the well-working of the organism as a whole," or again, "an activity of the living body in accordance with its specific excellences" (pp. 28-29).

3. The exceptions I am thinking of here include those instances when paternalistic interventions seem appropriate in medicine. See Gert and Culver (1976, 1979), Childress (1980), and Dworkin (1972). Goldblatt and I have defined a narrow range of medical problems ("acute, critical, easily treatable condi-

tions") which might exist as clinical medical problems even if competent patients declined medical intervention (Siegler and Goldblatt 1980).

4. It is illuminating to speculate on how much better Ivan Il'ich's medical care might have been had one or another of the four or five physicians he consulted from the onset of his disease until his death pursued this kind of analytic scheme. I am not suggesting that Il'ich's cancer could have been cured or alleviated by the medical techniques known to the nineteenth-century physicians. Rather, his clinical medical care could have been improved markedly if his physicians had been sensitive to such issues as why Il'ich presented to physicians when he did, and what factors—social, psychological, and personal, in addition to medical—were responsible for the generation and maintenance of his symptoms.

5. Feinstein's (1967) analysis of the strengths and limitations of modern medicine emphasizes the extraordinary importance of, and the successes of diagnostic evaluations based upon, the medical history. In terms of the data-gathering phase of the clinical evaluation, chapters 16 through 19 and 21 are particularly valuable. For example, in chapter 17, entitled "Art of Clinical Examination," Feinstein comments on history-taking as follows:

> History-taking, the most clinically sophisticated procedure of medicine, is an extraordinary investigative technique: in few other forms of scientific research does the observed object talk. The acquisition of data by this verbal process is far more complex than by the techniques of physician examination or of laboratory tests and the function of the history-taking apparatus cannot be learned from didactic lectures or textbooks. The student physician must be able to see and hear the subtle exchange of information in the intricate human relationship between patient and clinician ... (p. 299).

6. In this paper, I will not consider this important question, which is central to the practice of scientific clinical medicine. This issue relates to clinical judgment, the elaborate process of diagnosis, prognosis, and if appropriate, the institution of effective therapy, based upon established scientific principles. See Feinstein (1967, chap. 5, 13). At the conclusion of chapter 13, "The Objectives of Treatment," Feinstein writes:

> Although a clinician can be both a healer and a scientist, he cannot be an effective therapist if he merely joins these two roles in tandem by oscillating between them, adding laboratory science to bedside art. A clinician's objective in therapy is not just a conjunction, but a true synthesis of art and science, fusing the parts into a whole that unifies his work and makes his two roles one: a scientific healer. A clinician is always a healer; the healing function is basic to his care of sick people. The *scientific* performance of that function, however, is what distinguishes a well-trained medical or surgical clinician from other healers whose aid and comfort is given without the rational support of valid evidence, logical analysis, and demonstrable proofs (pp. 245-46).

7. "Self-abuse" is an elastic concept and may include a host of voluntary health risks ranging from participation in sports to failing to exercise. Other risks often included in this context are smoking, drinking alcohol to excess, using illicit or unnecessary drugs, being morbidly obese, failing to comply with prescribed medical regimens, and so forth.

8. The medical profession appears to have accepted the concept that physicians may decline to care for patients. For example, the 1957 version of the American Medical Association's *Principles of Medical Ethics* states: "A physician may choose whom he will serve. In an emergency, however, he should render service to the best of his ability" (sec. 5). I believe that the notion that physicians may choose whom they will serve first appeared in the AMA's 1912 revision of the *Principles of Medical Ethics*: "A physician is free to choose whom he will serve. He should, however, always respond to any request for his assistance in an emergency or whenever temperate public opinion expects the service" (chap. 1, sec. 4). This provision has been retained by the AMA's ad hoc Committee on Principles of Medical Ethics in the most recent proposed revision of the *Principles of Medical Ethics* (1979). Earlier AMA codes of medical ethics (1847 and 1903) and *Percival's Medical Ethics* (1803), from which the AMA's original code was derived, do not contain specific precedent for this principle. It would be valuable to review the legislative history of this provision of the 1912 revision of the AMA's *Principles of Medical Ethics* (see Percival, p. 258).

9. Physicians may occasionally disregard the law when they decide that certain patient needs require this action. This could be seen as a kind of conscientious objection to certain laws by the physician. In such cases the physician must be willing to assume certain risks and to accept potential consequences, voluntarily and conscientiously, presumably from a sense of overriding obligation to an individual patient. My point here is that physicians are not required to disobey the law and that it would not be appropriate for patients to demand that their physicians engage in illegal conduct. Conscientious objection to a statute cannot be demanded by a third party, in this instance, the patient (Childress 1979).

Bibliography

American Medical Association. 1847, 1903, 1912, 1957, 1979. *Principles of Medical Ethics*. Chicago: The American Medical Association.

Cassell, E.J. 1975. "Preliminary Explorations of Thinking in Medicine." *Ethics in Science and Medicine* 2: 1-12.

_____ . 1976. *The Healer's Art: A New Approach to The Doctor-Patient Relationship*. Philadelphia: J.B. Lippincott Co.

Childress, J.F. 1979. "Appeals to Conscience." *Ethics* 89: 315-35.

_____ . 1980. "Paternalism and Autonomy in Medical Decision Making." In *Frontiers in Medical Ethics: Applications in a Medical Setting*, edited by V. Abernethy. Cambridge, MA: Ballinger Publishing Co.

Dworkin, G. 1972. "Paternalism." *Monist* 56: 64-84.

Engel, G.L. 1977. "The Need for a New Medical Model: A Challenge for Bio-medicine." *Science* 196: 129-36.

Engelhardt, H.T., Jr. 1979. "Doctoring the Disease, Treating the Complaint, Helping the Patient: Some of the Works of Hygeia and Panacea." In *Knowing and Valuing: The Search for Common Roots*, edited by H.T. Engelhardt, Jr. and D. Callahan. Hastings-on-Hudson, NY: The Hastings Center.

Feinstein, A.R. 1967. *Clinical Judgment*. Baltimore: Williams and Wilkins Co.

Gert, B., and Culver, C.M. 1976. "Paternalistic Behavior." *Philosophy and Public Affairs* 6: 45-57.

_____ . 1979. "The Justification of Paternalism." *Ethics* 89: 199-210.

Groves, J.B. 1978. "Taking Care of the Hateful Patient." *New England Journal of Medicine* 298: 883-87.

Guttentag, O.E. 1978. "Care of the Healthy and the Sick from the Attending Physician's Perspective: Envisioned and Actual." In *Organism, Medicine, and Metaphysics*, edited by S.F. Spicker. Dordrecht, The Netherlands: D. Reidel Publishing Co.

_____ . 1985. "The Attending Physician as a Central Figure," pp. 107-126 in this volume.

Kass, L.R. 1975. "Regarding the End of Medicine and the Pursuit of Health." *The Public Interest* 40: 11-42.

Laín Entralgo, P. 1969. *Doctor and Patient.* Translated by F. Partridge. New York: McGraw-Hill Book Co.

Mechanic, D. 1978. *Medical Sociology.* 2d ed. New York: Free Press.

Merton, R.K. 1957. *Social Theory and Social Structure,* Rev. ed. New York: Free Press.

Parsons, T. 1951. *The Social System.* New York: Free Press.

Pellegrino, E.D. 1979. "The Anatomy of Clinical Judgments: Some Notes on Right Reason and Right Action," in *Clinical Judgment: A Critical Appraisal,* edited by H.T. Engelhardt, Jr., S.F. Spicker, and B. Towers. Dordrecht, The Netherlands: D. Reidel Publishing Co.

Percival, T. 1975 [1803]. *Percival's Medical Ethics.* Reprint edited by C.T. Leake. Huntington, NY: R.E. Krieger Publishing Co., 1975.

Plato. 1934. *The Laws.* Translated by A.E. Taylor. London: J.M. Dent and Sons.

Schaffner, K.F. 1979. "Commencement—1979." Address delivered at graduation exercises of the School of Medicine, University of Pittsburgh, June 1979.

Seldin, D.W. 1977. "The Medical Model: Bio-medical Science as the Basis of Medicine." In *Beyond Tomorrow: Trends and Prospects in Medical Science,* edited by Helene Jordon, New York: Rockefeller University Press.

Siegler, M., and Goldblatt, A.D. 1980. "Clinical Intuition: A Procedure for Balancing the Rights of Patients and the Responsibilities of Physicians." In *The Law-Medicine Relation: A Philosophical Exploration,* edited by S.F. Spicker, J.M. Healey, and H.T. Engelhardt, Jr. Dordrecht, The Netherlands: D. Reidel Publishing Co.

Szasz, T.S., and Hollender, M. 1956. "The Basic Models of the Doctor-Patient Relationship." *Archives of Internal Medicine* 97: 585-92.

Tolstoi, L.N. 1902. "The Death of Ivan Il'ich." In *More Tales from Tolstoi,* Translated by R. Nisbet Bain. London: Jarrold and Sons.

Tumulty, P.A. 1970. "What Is a Clinician and What Does He Do?" *New England Journal of Medicine* 283: 20-24.

Veatch, R.M. 1972. "Models for Ethical Medicine in a Revolutionary Age." *Hastings Center Report* 2: 5-7.

—————. 1973. "Generalization of Expertise." *Hastings Center Studies* 1: 29-40.

Modeling Clinical Medicine:
A Commentary on Mark Siegler

Kenneth F. Schaffner

Mark Siegler's paper reflects much of the spirit of Otto Guttentag's work. In his essay, Dr. Siegler, as Dr. Guttentag has done and has urged in the past, examines a key issue in medicine from the perspective of the attending physician. Siegler has also followed a type of pragmatic-phenomenological-existential method akin to the methodology that Dr. Guttentag has employed (Guttentag 1978). In my view, what Dr. Siegler has presented to us is a diachronic or temporally elaborated phenomenology of clinical practice. Previous analyses of the physician-patient relationship have usually been static, and not logical analyses of the temporally extended process.[1] These analyses, such as the well-known Szasz and Hollender (1956) model or the Veatch (1972) model, provide typologies, but lack the dynamic element necessary to capture the evolution and devolution found in all human relationships, and perhaps best seen in Siegler's novel notion of the doctor-patient accommodation. Siegler has provided us with a long overdue, sensitive, and thoughtful account of the clinical interaction.

The general thesis of my comments will be that it is important to supplement, in a synergistic manner, Siegler's diachronic phenomenological account with a more *theoretical* perspective on the nature of health and disease. Though I am in essential agreement with Siegler's position, I believe I can demonstrate that he tacitly subscribes to a theoretical model, in spite of his assertion that: "My concern is that these theoretical accounts of the nature and limits of clinical medicine never quite come to grips with the actualities of medical practice. I will therefore pursue a different program, beginning not with theories of health and disease, but rather with my own perception of how clinical medicine works in the realities of daily practice" (Siegler 1985, pp. 20-21).

I will proceed in two stages. First, I will need to develop a theoretical model of health and disease in the light of which I can present my general thesis concerning Siegler's essay. I will then consider in detail the four moments of Siegler's evolving doctor-patient relationship in the context of this model. The model which I shall elaborate in the next section owes much to the work of Drs. Eric Cassell (1976, chaps. 1-2) and George Engel (1960; 1977). This model was also stimulated by reflections on the thesis of Professors Gorovitz and MacIntyre (1976) that medicine is a "science of particulars," and by a close analysis of the nature of theory structure in the biomedical sciences (Schaffner 1980). I also believe it is foreshadowed in Dr. Guttentag's pioneering writings about the "clinical entity" (Guttentag 1949).

MEDICINE AS AN INTERLEVEL SCIENCE OF PARTICULARS

A theoretical model of health and disease, and also of the practice of medicine, will not only provide an appropriate context in which to comment on Dr. Siegler's essay; it will also permit me to address one of the themes which was proposed for the Conference on Changing Values in Medicine. In that context, Drs. Cassell and Siegler have suggested that "a reorientation of clinical practice from an activity almost solely based on the model of natural sciences, to one in which the *person-as-subject* becomes the primary scientific focus, will have a direct and pervasive impact on our understanding of clinical judgement and decision making" (brochure for the Conference on Changing Values in Medicine 1979, pp. 2-3).

Engel's Biopsychosocial Model

Over the past several decades, Dr. George Engel (1960, 1977) has been developing a biopsychosocial model of medicine. Engel contrasts this model with the current dominant biomedical model, which he construes both as reductionist and detrimental to the best interests of patients:

> The dominant model of disease today is biomedical, with molecular biology its basic scientific discipline. It assumes disease to be fully accounted for by deviations from the norm of measurable biological (somatic) variables. It leaves no room within its framework for the social, psychological, and behavioral dimensions of illness. The biomedical model not only requires that disease be dealt with as an entity independent of social behavior, it also demands that behavioral aberrations be explained on the basis of disordered somatic (biochemical or neurophysiological) processes. Thus the biomedical model embraces both reductionism, the philosophical view that complex phenomena are ultimately derived from a single primary principle, and mind-body dualism, the doctrine that separates the mental from the somatic (Engel 1977, p. 130).

The biopsychosocial model which Engel urges on the other hand is meant to supplement this current model which has taken on the status of an uncriticizable dogma. Engel notes the "enormous advantages of the biomedical approach," but also believes that "concentration on the biomedical and exclusion of the psychosocial distorts perspectives and even interferes with patient care" (p. 131). This supplementation and correction of the biomedical model involves

1. Recognition of complex causation: "The biomedical defect constitutes but one factor among many, the complex interaction of which
   ultimately may culminate in active disease or manifest illness ..."
   (p. 131).
2. Recognition of various levels of activity: "how [a disease such as
   diabetes with attendant polyuria, polydipsia, polyphagia, and
   weight loss, confirmed by laboratory documentation of relative
   insulin deficiency, is experienced, reported by, and affects any one
   individual requires] consideration of psychological, social and
   cultural factors, not to mention other concurrent or complicating
   biological factors" (p. 132).
3. Recognition of the individual variability of a disease, which "reflects
   as much ... [psychological, social, and cultural factors] as it does
   quantitative variations in the specific biochemical defect" (p. 132).

A biopsychosocial model "requires a scientifically rational approach to behavioral and psychosocial data for," as Engel notes, "these are the terms in which most clinical phenomena are reported by patients."[2] One needs such information to establish a clear relationship between particular biochemical processes and the *clinical* data of an illness.[3] Furthermore, Engel notes, "By evaluating *all* the factors contributing to both illness and patienthood, rather than giving primacy to biological factors alone, a biopsychosocial model would make it possible *to explain why* some individuals experience as 'illness' conditions which others regard merely as 'problems of living,' be they emotional reactions to life circumstances or somatic symptoms" (1977, p. 133, emphasis added). A biopsychosocial model thus should assist in accounting for "the dysphoria and the dysfunction which lead individuals to seek medical help, adopt the sick role, and accept the status of patienthood (Engel 1977, p. 133).

Engel's biopsychosocial model accordingly delineates a set of important and often overlooked considerations affecting our concepts of health, disease, and the role(s) of medicine. It seems to me, however, that the contrast which the model urges between the biomedical model and the biopsychosocial model is, on closer inspection, significantly less sharp than Engel suggests.

In my view, the problems Engel addresses are not so much due to the reliance on a biomedical model, which has reductionistic molecular biology as its basic scientific discipline, as they are conditioned by inaccurate perceptions of the nature of the biomedical sciences. The biomedical sciences in general, and molecular biology in particular, are usually seen through a lens fashioned by a universalist and unilevel construal of science, which is more appropriate for the physical and chemical sciences than it is for the life sciences. As both Engel and Cassell have noted in their writings, this distorted perception has powerful historical roots which it is mandatory to examine, even if only briefly, in order to diagnose the etiology of these problems and to correct our view of science. Such a correction is needed so that we may both retain the power over nature provided by the traditional reductionistic model of science, and at the same time develop a humanized model of clinical scientific medicine akin to the bio-psychosocial model, which is firmly grounded in the life sciences, and which focuses on the patient as an individual person with crucially important subjective features. As Dr. Siegler has noted in his essay, "most diagnoses, perhaps 70 to 90 percent, are made on the basis of the medical history" (p. 27). I think we need a diagnosis of this distorted perspective of biomedical science, as well as an overview history of science, to assist in the diagnosis as a prelude to therapy.

A Capsule History of Universalistic Biomedical Science

Much of the history of Western thought since the pre-Socratic philosophers, such as Thales, Heraclitus, Plato, and Aristotle, has been preoccupied with the search for universal truths. In Plato, individuals and particulars are pale, insubstantial shadows of universal forms: these universal forms are what are "really" real. In Aristotle, one finds a similar, though empirically modulated, search for the universal as the essence of science.[4]

This Greek legacy is still with us. In the Renaissance, the major works of Plato and Aristotle were rediscovered, and with Descartes, Leibniz, Galileo, and Newton, the search for and articulation of universal laws of the cosmos achieved stunning success, stimulating attempts to apply similar methods to biology and medicine. This approach, besides being universalist, was reductionistic (in the analytical sense), and also tended to be causally unifactorial.[5]

In the nineteenth century, the germ theory of disease was developed and brought into the mainstream of medicine by Pasteur, Lister, and Koch. Earlier in the same century, Rudolf Virchow applied the cell hypothesis of Schleiden and Schwann to pathology and proposed a cellular theory of disease. In the present century these approaches have been both amplified and deepened by the development of genetic and biochemical understandings of diseases.

What does this capsule history of science have to do with the problems of clinical medicine? My answer, partly paralleling that of Cassell

(1976, chap. 2), is that the magnificent successes of this "germ theory-cell theory" paradigm have tended to focus the clinician's attention on the universals—on diseases—and not on the actual particulars—the ill patients—that require the physician's help. Emphasis on the somatic or physical aspects of these universal pathological processes has also tended to oversimplify the physician's understanding of causality: the etiology of diseases presented in medical textbooks concentrates on the broad universal and often tends to neglect the fine structural details—the subtle complications and the intertwining multiple causal chains which arise from the interaction of the *disease* with the *host* or *patient* to produce the *illness*.[6]

Levels and Particularization

As one moves from the chemical sciences into the biological, one discovers that there are features that are present in living things that could be ignored in the nonliving domain. These features have led to vitalistic philosophies in the history of biomedical thought, but it is not on those that I want to concentrate. Rather, I want to emphasize two main characteristics that are encountered in this shift from the chemical to the biological; these two characteristics are further intensified as we move into the psychological and social sciences, and into the realm of human action, which includes an important normative or ethical dimension and is also the locus of the physician-patient interaction. These two characteristics are (1) levels of organization and (2) individuality. Levels of organization refers to the distinctions between the molecular level, the cellular level, the organ level, and the like. Individuality refers to the increasing differentiation that occurs due to complexity of structure, and the exposure of those structures to different environmental histories that condition each of them in different ways. In biology, it is already necessary to make use of *interlevel* theories and explanations; the most typically successful theories in immunology and genetics, for example, have parts that are drawn from several different levels of organization. To begin to discern universals in the special sense needed in biology and medicine, the biologist also already knows that, because of this developing individuality, he or she must attempt to control variation by careful selection of mutants or by extensive inbreeding to produce almost syngeneic experimental strains.

As examples of interlevel and individualized theories from biology, let us briefly consider the two-component theory of the immune response and the fine structure of mutants in the operon theory.

The so-called two-component theory of the immune response was first clearly articulated in the 1960s. The elements that constitute the theory are clearly multilevel, involving molecular entities (humoral antibodies), cells (stem cells and lymphocytes), tissues (peripheral lymphoid tissue), organs (thymus), and systems (the circulatory and lymph systems). The nature of the interaction among the components is clearly interlevel; for example, the thymus affects the developing stem cells, and T-cells (thymus-dependent cells) are known to regulate the amounts of antibody molecules produced by B-cells which mature into plasma cells. Figure 1 depicts this theory and the interactions.

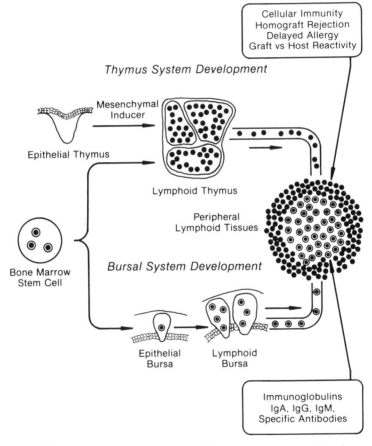

Figure 1. The two-component theory. "The two branches of the immune mechanism are believed to develop from the same lymphoid precursor. The central thymus system starts as an epithelial structure arising from third and fourth embryonic pharyngeal pouch and becomes a lymphoid organ under stimulation by a mesenchymal inducer. The bursal system develops by budding from the intestinal epithelium. After release from the central organs into the bloodstream, the lymphoid cells reassemble in peripheral lymphoid tissues. Here the lymphocytes—thymus dependent in origin—control cellular immunity, while bursa-dependent plasma cells synthesize serum antibodies" (fig. and legend from Good [1971, p. 9]. modified for reasons of space).

There is variation in this system from one species to another (e.g., birds have a well-defined bursa whereas mammals do not), and there is extensive individual variation among humans, from subtle differences in responses to allergens to more extreme congenital problems, such as the Di George syndrome in which some babies are born without a thymus. These individuals have a functional antibody-producing system but are not able to develop a homograft response.

More striking variation in a system that has been studied down to the molecular level is found in the operon theory of genetic regulation in the common intestinal bacterium *Escherichia Coli.* This theory is also multilevel as regards its components; for example, it initially postulated both genes and chemically characterized substances (mRNA), but its primary interest to us lies in the extraordinary amount of variation detectable within one type of mutation of the system. In the operon theory in its classical *lac* form,[7] regulation takes place via synthesis of a proteinaceous *repressor* which, in the absence of an exogenous *inducer*, binds to the *operator* gene preventing transcription of the structural genes controlled by the operator. (The complex consisting of operator and controlled structural genes is termed the *operon*.) A well-known operator gene mutation that prevents repressor binding is known as an operator constitutive mutation (O^c). A careful fine-structure analysis of this "one type" of mutation by Smith and Sadler (1971) has disclosed that some 590 different subtypes of O^c mutation are characterizable.

The philosophical points to stress here are that biological theories already (1) reflect the need to gather data from several levels, and (2) contain sufficient variation within them that a simple universal generalization will not capture the properties in any facile way.[8]

In medicine, as George Engel has stressed, the psychological and social levels of reality also affect the patient. A satisfactory diagnosis, etiology, and prognosis will often have to take account of not only chemical and cellular features, but it will also need to gather information from these higher levels. This multilevel information is also likely to contain highly individual elements. In medical textbooks and journal articles discussing diseases and reporting new clinical investigations, "the individuality is often filtered out, usually employing a statistical methodology. What is left are important multilevel generalizations, absolutely necessary for medical science that *then* have to be *reindividualized* by the physician (Schaffner 1979). Part of this reindividualization may require drawing on levels of generalization which are not usually considered part of medicine, such as family interactions. Ethical principles may be required to assist and clarify decision choices guiding diagnoses and treatments where costs and risks to the patient are involved. Again, it is the *disease* which is individualized in the patient which constitutes the *illness* the physician must treat.

Such considerations as why the patient became ill; the specific nature of the patient's somatic and psychological defenses; the best course of therapy for that person in his or her individual circumstances of history, habits, lifestyle, emotions, employment, family, and friends; and the sensitivity to incorporating that information, are foreign to a preoccupation with broad universals and with a concentration on the somatic components typified by a cellular pathology. Lest I be misinterpreted, I must emphasize that cellular pathology, antibody titers, and the like, are crucially important components used in clinical decision making; but they are components or partial elements in the constellation of an illness.

This point can be illustrated in two reasonably typical diseases. A review of the principal mechanisms operative in congestive heart failure discloses the role of interlevel interactions in this disease, from the atomic (sodium ions) through the cellular and organ interactions to the role of whole body exercise and emotional excitement. These interactions are depicted in Figure 2.

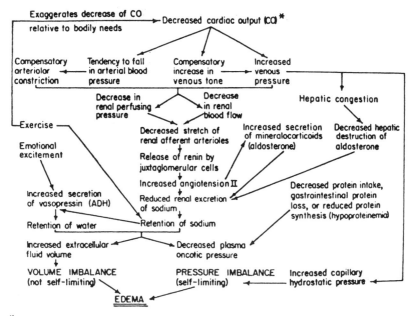

*
In high output failure (hyperthyroidism, anemia) the CO is elevated but still relatively insufficient to meet bodily needs

Figure 2. Schematic diagram of the principal mechanisms operating in congestive heart failure. Detweiler, 1977.

The need to be sensitive to finer and finer subclasses (at least some of which are slices from an almost continuous spectrum) of a disease is typified in individuals suffering from a form of systemic lupus erythematosus which affects the kidney. Systemic lupus erythematosus (sometimes known as lupus or SLE) is a chronic inflammatory disease which affects a wide variety of organ systems including skin, joints, hematologic and nervous systems, and the kidneys. It is at least partially an autoimmune disease in which the body's immune system turns against itself. It has been proposed by Dixon (1971) and others that the patient's own DNA may act as an antigen, stimulating antibodies with which the DNA makes complexes, which in turn binds complement, initiating active polymorphonuclear leukocytes to release proteolytic enzymes, which "chew up" the kidney's basement membrane.

Even if the general pathogenesis (though not the specific etiology) is clear, the nature of the disease is very variable, waxing and waning and manifesting itself in protean forms. Even in the subcategory on which I am focusing, lupus-kidney or lupus nephritis, there are some five different sub-subtypes which in reality lie partially on a multidimensional spectrum (see Table 1). Treatment will vary depending on the subclass, and the treatment modality may have to be shifted quickly if the patient moves from one subclass to another, such as from diffuse proliferative lupus nephritis to late stage lupus nephropathy. In making these clinical decisions regarding therapy, the physician has to gather evidence from a variety of levels and also has to keep the history of the patient in mind.

What I have tried to show in this excursion into a biopsychosocial model is that medicine must, if it is to be faithful to its scientific basis, be both concerned with interlevel interactions and also sensitive to individual variations. In the next section I shall return to specific comments on Dr. Siegler's paper and attempt to show how he *implicitly* accepts some of these features, and also how his diachronic phenomenological account of the doctor-patient interaction synergistically extends some of the facets of this elaborated biopsychosocial model.

SIEGLER'S FOUR CLINICAL MOMENTS
OF THE PHYSICIAN-PATIENT INTERACTION

One major theme of Siegler's analysis of the evolving doctor-patient relationship is what philosophers might characterize as its "conventionalistic" character.[9] Siegler writes that "the nature of clinical medicine is not an entity to be discovered like a truth of nature, but that it is *defined and created* in the context of a doctor-patient accommodation. There is no single 'nature of clinical medicine,' but many such natures" (p. 21, emphasis added).

Table 1. Clinical-Morphologic Classification of Lupus Nephritis*

	Focal Proliferative	Diffuse Proliferative	Membranous	Mesangial	Late Stage "Nephropathy"
Hypertension	none	most; occasionally severe	occasional	none	all; severe
Urinalysis					
Rbc	70%	100%	50%	minimal	occasional
Protein	100%	100%	100%	minimal	100%
Nephrotic Syndrome	rare	50%	50-80%	none	some
Serum Creatinine	rarely abnormal	most elevated	occasionally severe	occasional mild elevation	all elevated
Course: Remission	usual	½, but ¼ relapse	1/3; relapse common	almost all	none
Progression	none	½, often rapid	1/3, slow	only with transition	slow
Transition	rare to diffuse proliferative	with remission only to membranous or mesangial	rarely to diffuse proliferative	not infrequent to diffuse proliferative or membranous	none
Five-Year Mortality	30%	70%	30%	unknown	100% unless dialysis or transplantation

*From Medsger, 1979, after Baldwin et al., 1977, and Fries et al., 1974

My thesis is that (1) this definitional and creative element is significantly less pervasive than Dr. Siegler maintains, and (2) an analysis of Siegler's arguments in light of the elaborated biopsychosocial model developed above points to the sources of biological, psychological, social, and ethical factors which govern and constrain the evolving doctor-patient relationship. I shall develop these positions by reviewing in sequence Siegler's four moments: (1) the prepatient phase; (2) the initial encounter of the patient with the physician; (3) the doctor-patient accommodation; and (4) the doctor-patient relationship.

The Prepatient Phase

Siegler eloquently describes how Tolstoi depicts the process by which Ivan Il'ich first becomes a patient. As he notes, "the decision to seek medical counsel was reached because Ivan Il'ich had a sense of not feeling well and because his wife urged him to seek medical attention and cure" (p. 25). Dr. Siegler stresses that "Ivan Il'ich and his wife were not identifying the pain, or bad taste, or loss of appetite as the illness; instead they were focusing on his irritability and ill temper and the impact of these on the family's tranquility. It appears that Ivan Il'ich sought medical attention because of the influence of his family—his wife's urging—and perhaps because entering the medical system offered a potentially extenuating excuse for his aberrant behavior" (p. 25).

It seems to me that this illustration supports exactly the biopsychosocial model described above. We have an instance of complex causation with biomedical, psychological, familial, and social (i.e., adoption of the "sick role") factors, which collectively generate and identify the "iatrotropic stimulus."

The Initial Encounter: Data Gathering and Data Reduction

Dr. Siegler characterizes the second clinical moment of the doctor-patient encounter as one in which there are two intertwined components. In the first of these components, the clinician determines the nature of the iatrotropic stimulus,[10] whether the problem is a medical one, and whether the patient will be a "good patient" or a "problem patient." In the second and usually inseparable component, the physician applies the clinical method with its two subcomponents, data gathering and data reduction.

This phase is usually thought to be the most scientific and objective phase of the doctor-patient encounter. Dr. Guttentag (1960), following von Gebsattel (1954), refers to it as the stage of "estrangement: the objective scientific stage."

But as Siegler points out, this second clinical moment involves complex and subtle verbal and paraverbal exchanges: "an enormous amount of human and personal interaction is occurring between patient and doctor" (p. 28). Even in the data reduction stage in which a diagnosis and a differential diagnosis are generated, emphasis is on the individual patient and not on general theories of pathophysiology.

Again, it appears that the elaborated biopsychosocial model is being instantiated in Siegler's second moment. Emphasis is on communication and on data from all levels, including the behavioral and the quasi-ethical levels (as in the "good patient"). The significance of the individual illness rather than the general disease is implicitly stressed by Siegler. Accordingly, it appears that a further elaboration of the tenets of the theoretical model discussed above can assist in clarifying important parts of this moment.

The Doctor-Patient Accommodation and the
Doctor-Patient Relationship

The third of Dr. Siegler's clinical moments is the one on which he places most emphasis. It is in this stage of the evolving patient-physician encounter that "the nature of clinical medicine is defined and created in the context of this [doctor-patient] accommodation, which must be mutually agreed upon by both participants" (pp. 28-29). There is, however, no sharp line of demarcation between the third moment of the clinical encounter and the fourth stage, the achievement of a doctor-patient relationship. Siegler suspects that "the essential feature of a doctor-patient relationship is the exchange of a deep bond of trust between patient and doctor" (p. 34). However, he also notes that "the doctor-patient accommodation and the doctor-patient relationship are always in a state of dynamic equilibrium; mutual trust tends to drive the equation toward maintaining the doctor-patient relationship, but new circumstances constantly force the patient and physician to reassess the stability of their ongoing medical relationship" (p. 35). These new circumstances, Siegler notes, can be changes in the patient on either the biomedical level (new disease) or the psychological level (new attitudes or new demands). The altered circumstances can also arise because of changes in the physician, e.g., a change in specialization or physician attitudes.

I believe that the doctor-patient accommodation and the catalytic effect of "trust," which in Siegler's dynamic model drives the accommodation to the status of a relationship, can be usefully augmented by further development of a biopsychosocial model of medicine.[11] I would suggest that the dynamic processes occurring in the accommodation are both (1) interactions *among* various levels described in the biopsychosocial model, and (2) very special and complex interactions which occur in the social and ethical levels of exchange. The net process intertwining the descriptive and the norma- tive is reminiscent of Rawls's process of arriving at a position of "re- flective equilibrium" (1971, p. 20). Further analysis of this process by Norman Daniels (1979) and others[12] indicates that the process is extremely complex. Daniels writes:

> Arguments [to a position of reflective equilibrium], however, can be viewed as inferences from a number of relevant background theories, in particular, from a theory of the person, a theory of procedural justice, general social theory, and a theory of the role of morality in society (including the ideal of a well-ordered society). These *level* III theories, as I shall call them, are what persuade us to adopt the contract apparatus, with all its constraints (call it the *level* II apparatus). Principles chosen at *level* II are subject to two constraints: (i) they must match our considered moral judgments in (partial) reflective equilibrium; and (ii) they must yield a feasible, stable, well-ordered society. I will call *level* I the partial reflective equilibrium that holds between the moral principles and the relevant set of considered moral judgments. *Level* IV contains the body of social theory relevant to testing *level* I principles (and *level* III theories) for "feasibility" (p. 260).

Dr. Siegler's description of the process of the doctor-patient accom- modation and its deepening into the doctor-patient relationship, as well as the illustration of the pregnant woman with psoriasis, sup- port the interpretation. The doctor-patient relationship is affected and constrained both by the physician's and patient's values and partic- ular circumstances. When these various multilevel, multifactorial, and highly individual elements are acknowledged, I doubt there is as much free play in the relationship as Siegler suggests through which definition and creativity can exercise their influence. However, the acknowledgment of such factors does not negate Dr. Siegler's superb and sensitive analysis; rather it indicates the manner in which we may begin to come to a deeper understanding of this very complex and important human interaction: the doctor-patient relationship.

Notes

1. The only exceptions of which I am aware are von Gebsattel (1954) and Guttentag (1960), who uses von Gebsattel.

2. See Engel and Morgan's (1969) detailed account interdigitating a scientific approach to patient interviewing and clinical diagnosis.

3. As both Engel (1977) and Feinstein (1967) have noted, biochemical "abnormalities" may be present without producing clinical manifestations, and vice versa.

4. Compare Gorovitz and MacIntyre (1976), Lescher (1973), and Hintikka (1972) for discussions of universality in Aristotelian science. (I thank James Lennox for these last two references.)

5. Compare Engel (1977, p. 131).

6. Compare Feinstein (1967, pp. 24-25).

7. See Strickberger (1976, chap. 29) for a clear discussion of the various types of operons, including the *lac* form.

8. The variation involves polytypic overlapping and not simply an "average." See Guttentag (1949) and Schaffner (1980) for a distinction between "mean" and "type."

9. *Conventionalistic* is being used in the sense employed by Poincaré (1905), namely, definitions which appear to play more than a definitional role.

10. The term *iatrotropic stimulus* is, as Siegler notes, to be attributed to Feinstein. Curiously, unlike Feinstein (1967, pp. 144-45), Siegler does not stress that what is usually termed the *chief complaint* is often not identical to the iatrotropic stimulus.

11. Though I cannot develop the point in this essay, it seems to me that the notion of "trust" could be further analyzed to determine which factors in the doctor-patient relationship generate and sustain trust. An examination of Parsons's (1951) social analysis of the relationship suggests that "universalism, functional specificity, and affective neutrality" are important factors. Each of these factors, however, needs to be scrutinized and related to Siegler's account and to the biopsychosocial model and would exceed the scope of these comments.

12. See the essays by Ronald Dworkin, R.M. Hare, Joel Feinberg, and David Lyons in Daniels's (1976) anthology on Rawls.

Bibliography

Baldwin, D.G., Gluck, M.C., Lowenstein, J., and Gallo, G.R. 1974. "Lupus Nephritis: Clinical Course as Related to Morphological Forms and their Transitions." *American Journal of Medicine* 62: 12-20.

Cassell, E.J. 1976. *The Healer's Art: A New Approach to the Doctor-Patient Relationship.* Philadelphia: J.B. Lippincott Co.

Daniels, N. 1979. "Wide Reflective Equilibrium and Theory Acceptance in Ethics." *Journal of Philosophy* 76: 256-82.

Daniels, N., ed. 1976. *Reading Rawls.* New York: Basic Books.

Detweiler, J.C. 1977. "Cardiac Drugs." In *Veterinary Pharmacology and Therapeutics*, edited by L. Jones, N.H. Booth, and L.F. McDonald, 4th ed. Ames: Iowa State University Press.

Dixon, F. 1971. "Glomerulonephritis and Immunopathology." In *Immunobiology*, edited by R.A. Good and D.W. Fisher. Stamford, CT: Sinauer Associates.

Engel, G.L. 1960. "A Unified Concept of Health and Disease." *Perspectives in Biology and Medicine* 3: 459-85.

————. 1977. "The Need for a New Biomedical Model: A Challenge for Biomedicine." *Science* 196: 129-36.

Engel, G.L., and Morgan, W.L., Jr. 1969. *The Clinical Approach to Patient.* Philadelphia: W.B. Saunders.

Feinstein, A.R. 1967. *Clinical Judgment.* Baltimore: Williams and Wilkins.

Fries, J.F., Powers, R., and Kempson, R.L. 1974. "Late-Stage Lupus Nephropathy." *Journal of Rheumatology* 1:2: 166-75.

Good, R.A. 1971. "Disorders of the Immune System." In *Immunobiology*, edited by R.A. Good and D.W. Fisher. Stamford, CT: Sinauer Associates.

Gorovitz, S., and MacIntyre, A. 1976. "Toward a Theory of Medical Fallibility." *Journal of Medicine and Philosophy* 1: 51-64.

Guttentag, O.E. 1949. "On the Clinical Entity." *Annals of Internal Medicine* 31: 484-96.

_____ . 1960. "A Course Entitled 'The Medical Attitude': An Orientation in the Foundations of Medical Thought." *Journal of Medical Education* 35: 903-07.

_____ . 1978. "Care of the Healthy and the Sick from the Attending Physician's Perspective: Envisioned and Actual." In *Organism, Medicine, and Metaphysics*, edited by S.F. Spicker. Dordrecht, The Netherlands: D. Reidel Publishing Co.

_____ . 1985. "The Attending Physician as a Central Figure," pp. 107-126 in this volume.

Hintikka, J. 1972. "On the Ingredients of an Aristotelian Science." *Nous* 6: 65-98.

Lescher, J. 1973. "Aristotle on Form, Substance, and Universals: A Dilemma." *Phronesis* 30: 169-79.

Medsger, T.A., Jr. 1979. "An Approach to Lupus Nephritis." Address delivered to the Conference on Systemic Lupus Erythematosus, University of Pittsburgh, March 1979.

Parsons, T. 1951. *The Social System.* New York: Free Press.

Poincaré, H. 1905. *Science and Hypothesis.* Translated by G.B. Halsted. New York: Science Press.

Rawls, J. 1971. *A Theory of Justice.* Cambridge, MA: Harvard University Press.

Schaffner, K.F. 1979. "Commencement—1979." Address delivered at graduation exercises of the School of Medicine, University of Pittsburgh, June 1979.

_____ . 1980. "Theory Structure in the Biomedical Sciences." *Journal of Medicine and Philosophy* 5: 57-97.

Siegler, M. 1985. "The Nature and Limits of Clinical Medicine," pp. 19-41 in this volume.

Smith, T.F., and Sadler, J.R. 1971. "The Nature of Lactose Operator Constitutive Mutations." *Journal of Molecular Biology* 59: 273-305.

Strickberger, M.W. 1976. *Genetics.* 2d edition. New York: Macmillan Publishing Co.

Szasz, T., and M. Hollender. 1956. "The Basic Models of the Doctor-Patient Relationship." *Archives of Internal Medicine* 97: 585-92.

Veatch, R.M. 1972. "Models for Ethical Medicine in a Revolutionary Age." *Hastings Center Report* 2: 5-7.

von Gebsattel, V.F. 1954. *Prolegomena einer Medizinischen Anthropologie.* Berlin: Springer.

Causation and the Locus
of Medical Intervention

Stephen Toulmin

The aim of the present paper is to reactivate our sense of what *medical causation* implied before the rise of twentieth-century "scientific medicine," and to show that the new dependence of medical techniques on scientific research has not materially changed these considerations and relations.

THE EVERYDAY CONCEPT OF CAUSATION

We may begin by considering a sample, everyday situation that illustrates the force and implications of causal issues and diagnoses. Consider, for instance, a first scenario:

It is midsummer. The child has been given a new toy as a birthday gift. It is a kind of erector set designed on the same principles as card castles. The point is to build up as many units as possible into a "castle" without destroying the equilibrium of the whole structure. Since the child is only nine, it finds this task tricky, and can rarely place more than a dozen units so that they stand without falling. On this occasion sixteen units are already in place; but when the seventeenth is placed in position, the whole castle collapses.

The child is frustrated: "Oh, Dad, must you keep walking around like that? You're shaking the table!"; or else, "Can't we have the window shut? The draft blows everything over!"

Mother intervenes, saying, "Don't let it upset you, darling! You'll get better at it with practice"; and adding, in an aside to Father, "It's a silly game anyway—I can't think why your sister got it for him. Really, the Federal Trade Commission ought to keep a sharper eye on toy advertisements."

The question, "What made the child's castle fall down?", may thus be met in practice by responses of several different kinds, each of which operates on its own distinct level. Even as it stands, for instance, our scenario implies six such responses:

—"The seventeenth unit upset the equilibrium."

—"Father's heavy footfall shook the table."

—"There was a draft from the window."

—"The game calls for more dexterity than so young a child possesses."

—"It's a silly game anyway."

—"The FTC doesn't monitor the toy industry closely enough."

Nor, given the varied standpoints of the different participants in this scenario, can it be conclusively argued that any one of these responses points to the one and only relevant (meaningful, correct, true) cause of the castle's collapse. On the contrary, from one point of view or another, each of these responses is a relevant and meaningful response; and, on occasion, all of these responses might even turn out to be true at the same time.

With this first scenario fresh in our minds, we may notice five preliminary points about the everyday concept of causation:

(1) *Causes are ways of effecting outcomes.* If we speak of the collapse of the child's castle as an "effect," we treat its occurrence (or nonoccurrence) as something that could in principle be "effected," that is, brought about. To inquire, "What made the castle fall down?", thus raises the question of how this occurrence could have been produced, or prevented, by outside (specifically, by human) intervention. If an effective possible intervention is recognized and agreed upon— if it is agreed, that is, who or what was responsible for the castle's collapse—then we have arrived at a strong candidate for the title of "cause" of the collapse. The cause of the castle's falling down is the means whereby this outcome might be (and presumably was) brought about; and the question, "What caused the castle to fall down?", is thus to be construed as meaning, "What crucial intervening factor brought this outcome about?"

(2) *There are always multiple possible causes of any occurrence.* In dealing with questions of causation, there is from the outset an evident difference between our apparent expectations and our actual practice. We commonly tend to talk about causation in singular terms: referring to the crucial intervening factor in any situation as the cause of the corresponding occurrence (or effect), so implying that one and only one such intervening factor must have been the crucial one. Yet, as our scenario illustrates, everyday questions about causation can frequently be given multiple responses, all of them more or less relevant and meaningful. How are we to reconcile our expectations with our practice? The answer is: we always address questions about causation from particular standpoints. Different participants in any situation address questions of causation with different interests in mind, have access to (or power over) different variables in the situation, and regard

different features in the situation as open to change, either by themselves or by others. From its own standpoint, the child understand-
ably takes the playability of the game for granted and looks for the
cause of the castle's collapse in external agents or factors, for example, Father or the draft. By contrast, Mother's view reaches further,
to embrace also the aunt who sent the game as a gift, the firm that
manufactured it, and the Federal Trade Commission that permitted
it to be marketed and advertised as it was. (The child probably does
not know that the FTC even exists!)

(3) *Causation is not the same as causality.* The practical ways in
which we talk and think about causes and effects in everyday life
need to be distinguished from the theoretical ways in which natural
scientists talk and think about "mechanisms," "fields," and other such
explanatory factors in accounting for natural phenomena. In particular, scientists demand a kind of consensus about the correct scientific
explanation of any natural phenomenon that is rarely available when
we are asking what agent or factor was crucially responsible for some
untoward occurrence. If we seek a theoretical understanding of all
that is scientifically involved in the success or failure of the child's
efforts at building up a castle, this will lead us to explore the physics
of the situation. So far as physics goes, however, there is nothing
to choose between the castle's staying up and its falling down; these
are simply two out of many possible natural sequences, all of them
equally intelligible in physical terms. An exhaustive scientific account
of the child's situation will thus identify all of the varied physical
factors and conditions involved that may conceivably be relevant to
the outcome of the child's efforts; and, for these purposes, it will not
be necessary to raise questions about causation at all.

This is not to say that the notions of causation and causality are
entirely unconnected. On the contrary, knowing what factors and
conditions are causally relevant to any happening (in the causality
sense) allows us to identify *possible* causes of that occurrence (in the
causation sense). A complete physical representation of the child's
situation, for instance, will draw our attention to all of the potential
causes of different possible outcomes; but the factors in question can
be regarded as *actually* causative or efficacious only if we go beyond
what physics tells us and make the further, nonscientific judgment
by which prime significance, or responsibility, is attributed to one
or another factor, in the light of our entire practical understanding
of the situation concerned.

(4) *Questions about causation directly raise issues of responsibility.*
In thinking about the everyday notions of cause and effect, the role
of causation in the law is a better object of comparison than the role
of causality in natural science. Suppose that a house catches fire under

suspicious circumstances. The judge's responsibility will be to answer the question, "What caused this event?" From the standpoint of the law, the meaning of that question is: "What agent, action, or agency is to be held responsible for that event?" In judicial practice, that is to say, the standing presumption is that houses catch fire only in consequence of specific agencies—including, of course, both acts of commission, such as arson, and acts of omission, such as failing to extinguish a cigarette butt. (Even where natural processes bring about the same outcomes, e.g., when a house is set on fire by lightning, the courts still traditionally use the language of agency, attributing such events to acts of God.) Convincing attributions of responsibility will frequently require us, of course, to draw on our scientific understanding of the processes involved. But such a diagnosis will itself come under the heading of applied science, mobilizing our prior scientific understanding to shed light on one particular practical situation. And it is on the practical place that issues of causation are most naturally and literally at home. In the courts, as in everyday life, the question is, "Was there anybody whose action or failure to act might have produced or prevented the specific outcome under consideration? If so, who?"

(5) *Different standpoints presuppose different modes of intervention.* Suppose that we look at the six alternative responses to the question, "What made the child's castle fall down?" As we move down our list—beginning with the child's immediate action of putting the seventeenth unit into position, and proceeding step by step to the Federal Trade Commission's responsibility for monitoring toy advertisements—we broaden our view at each stage to include a progressively larger constellation of factors and agents. Correspondingly, at each stage we free up for consideration, as possible villains in the case, factors hitherto taken for granted or even concealed; and, in this way, we open up the possibility of producing or preventing the outcome in question by broader (even, by more "radical") modes of intervention.

To begin with, we may say: "The manner in which the child added the seventeenth unit destroyed the equilibrium." By doing so, we place responsibility for the collapse squarely on the child, implying that, without any other changes, it could have positioned the seventeenth unit differently and so have prevented the collapse. By contrast, the child may say: "Father's heavy footfall (or the draft from the window) did it." This alternative response requires us to broaden our view to include the room in which the child is building its castle. By pointing to Father or the draft, the child shifts the burden of responsibility: at the cost of some inconvenience (given the summer heat) Father or the whole family could have acted in ways that would have enabled the child to add more pieces without catastrophe, and so postponed the collapse. In turn, Mother broadens the perspective still further: she sees that the collapse, and the child's consequent frustration, might have been obviated if only the gift had been held back until the child was older—or else, if the toy had never been put on the market at all, or if it had, at least been advertised in more appropriate language. In this way, she shifts responsibility again: to Auntie, the manufacturers, or the FTC.

How, then, do we choose in practice between different possible responses to questions about causation? We do so by asking ourselves who exactly, in that situation, had the most obvious power to alter the eventual outcome, had a consequent duty of care, and so should have acted differently. In answering that question, we may take a very narrow view: the child should have placed the seventeenth unit more carefully. Or we may take a somewhat broader view: Auntie should have waited a couple of years before giving the child this particular present. Or we can take a comprehensive, sociopolitical view: the FTC should have enforced stricter policies. As a result, there is a direct relationship between the standpoint from which we view questions about causation, the kinds of actions we are ready to regard as causes, and the loci at which we regard it as appropriate to intervene, so as to bring about (or prevent) outcomes of the kind in question.

CAUSATION IN THE MEDICAL CONTEXT

The points that the first scenario brings to light can also be applied to examples from medicine. Consider, for instance, a second scenario:

It is early morning. After a restless night, the businessman wakes with acute stomach pains, and the dark color of his feces indicates internal bleeding. "Oh, Lord!" he says to his wife. "I don't know what you gave me for dinner last night, but my ulcers are certainly acting up."

A visit to the doctor confirms his fears: his ulcerated digestive tract is reacting acutely to some insult. "I've told you my opinion before," says the doctor. "The stresses and frustrations of your present job are too severe for a perfectionist like you. You would do your digestion a good turn if you found a different position; but meanwhile you'll have to be extra careful about your diet."

Back home the wife is on the telephone to her best friend: "Poor Jim! The soup was too rich for his delicate stomach. Still, I can't stand the way the firm takes advantage of him. If the management were only reorganized, Jim would be under less pressure, and I'm sure he wouldn't have so much stomach trouble. What is it about the way industry is organized nowadays? It takes a terrible toll on people in executive positions."

The question, "What caused the businessman's symptoms?", can be met once again by responses of several different kinds, each of which operates on a different level. To list six possible responses:

—"Last night's dinner triggered off the symptoms."
—"His wife spiced the soup too richly."
—"His ulcers are acting up."
—"He's too much of a perfectionist to stand the stress of his present job."
—"The executives in this firm live one hell of a life."
—"Present-day industrial organization exposes middle management to great stress."

As before, no argument requires us to say that one and only one of these responses is uniquely relevant (meaningful, correct, true). From one standpoint or another, each of the responses may be entirely appropriate; and, on occasion, all of them may turn out to be true at the same time.

To go further: (1) If we speak of the businessman's symptoms as being effects, we treat their occurrence (or nonoccurrence) as outcomes that could be effected (i.e., brought about) or prevented by specific kinds of antecedent interventions. If things had gone differently beforehand, then the symptoms would simply not have appeared. The question, "What caused them?" accordingly means: "What crucial factor or action, from among the antecedent conditions, brought about these symptoms as its specific outcome?"

(2) Once again, the multiple responses available to this causal question reflect the multiple standpoints from which the symptoms can legitimately be viewed, according to the specific interests and attitudes of the particular onlooker or participant involved. Should we label the spicy soup as the cause and so point a finger at the wife? Should we take on the ulcers themselves and so question the doctor's treatment? Or should we bring in the firm's organization and so play social critics? The chosen response depends on the questioner's stake in the situation, the variables that he or she has power over or access to, and the features that he or she accepts as open to change in practice. The businessman is interested only in alleviating his complaint without changing his style of life; the doctor shifts attention away from the ulcers and raises questions about the businessman's job; the wife has her own (ambiguous) standpoint, alternately blaming herself for the immediate crisis and criticizing the firm (or the entire industrial system) for her husband's general problem.

(3) As before, however, all these causal questions have to do with causation—and so with responsibility—rather than with causality, that is, with scientific explanation. Physiology gives us an understanding of the causality of digestion, that is, of all the different factors and conditions that can potentially serve as causes in our diagnoses of particular digestive disorders. But these factors and conditions can

operate actually as causes only within particular situations and on particular occasions; to pick any one of them out as the cause is then to see it as standing out from the entire concatenation of physiological relationships, as being of crucial significance in this particular case for this particular diagnosis. The presence of an ulcer in somebody's digestive tract, for instance, will become a cause if, on some particular occasion, the rest of the situation enables the ulcer to make its presence known by generating symptoms. But picking and choosing between the different factors and conditions, and identifying any one or two of those factors and conditions as "causative," takes us beyond physiology into clinical medicine proper; it takes us, also, beyond the realm of physiological causality (and pure science) into the realm of practical causation (and applied science).

(4) Thus, questions of medical causation do not raise intellectual questions about scientific explanation as much as they do practical questions about the attribution of responsibility. In deciding what factors were causative, in the context of a practical diagnosis, we make assumptions about the locus of responsibility—about whose actions, or failures to act, can be held responsible for the symptoms under consideration—and also about the available ("effectable") modes of intervention for dealing with the symptoms or preventing their recurrence. To spell out this particular aspect of the issue: "Is there any identifiable agent or agents whose actions or omissions can be held responsible for the businessman's pain and bleeding? If so, who? If not, how else could those symptoms have occurred?"

(5) Finally, then, how do we decide which of the alternative responses to the question, "What caused the businessman's symptoms?", to focus on? Suppose that we look at the alternative responses in turn; and suppose that we start from last night's dinner and proceed step by step to the doctor, the firm, and the industrial system. At each step, we broaden our view to include a larger constellation of factors and agents as possible causes—that is, as possible targets for the attribution of responsibility. At each stage, correspondingly, we free up for consideration factors hitherto taken for granted or even concealed; and, in doing so, we open up the possibility that such outcomes might be most effectively changed by broader (or more "radical") kinds of interventions.

Focusing on the immediate collision between last night's dinner and the businessman's ulcerated tract is like focusing on the child's positioning of the seventeenth unit. It narrows our vision and places the responsibility solely on the businessman himself: if only he had eaten more prudently he could have avoided this attack. To blame the symptoms on the spiciness of the soup, by contrast, shifts the burden of responsibility to his wife; by taking more care with the condiments, she might have spared him a recurrence of his standing digestive trouble. Pointing directly at the ulcers widens our view further by indicating another possible locus of intervention: if only the businessman's physician or surgeon eliminated the ulcers from his digestive tract he could eat with greater freedom even while keeping his present job. As for the doctor, he broadens the issue further by raising the legitimate question as to whether the businessman is not himself responsible for the continuation of his trouble and also the person who could best remedy it—if only he heeded the doctor's advice and switched to a more suitable job. The wife's telephone conversation opens up the possibility of yet broader interventions: maybe the firm should intervene to spare its executives avoidable stress; or maybe the whole competitive industrial bureaucracy needs reorganizing so as to stop exposing executives to damaging conditions of work.

RESPONSIBILITY AND THE MEDICAL PROFESSION

These two scenarios were designed to draw attention to a particular set of relationships. In the current age of scientific medicine, we have been tempted to assume that questions of practical causation in medicine have the same unambiguous force and status that we associate with issues of scientific causality in, for example, physiology. Instead, issues of medical causation raise the same ambiguous questions—about responsibility, failure to act, contributory negligence, and the rest— that one associates rather with judicial issues of causation, civil liability, and criminal responsibility. This change of perspective has important consequences for our understanding of the scope of medical responsibility, to which we must turn next.

People have often been tempted to suppose that the "scientific" physician should view all his cases from the single, unambiguous standpoint of "science." To accept that conclusion, however, would mean placing arbitrary limitations on the physician's attention and subjecting his clinical judgment to a kind of tunnel vision. Medicine, like law, is a practical enterprise; the causal questions that arise within any practical enterprise are never free of ambiguity. They can always be raised from a variety of standpoints and dealt with by different kinds of interventions, some of them local and immediate, others involving larger scale actions and changes. Accordingly, as in any practical enterprise, the ways in which medical causation is discussed reflect current assumptions about responsibility for bringing about or preventing medical outcomes, and thus current views about the acceptable and effective loci of intervention. The thrust of the present argument is that current ideas about the acceptable loci of intervention are restricted by implicit assumptions about the proper scope of medical practice and limitations of the physician's professional role.

How do these restrictions show themselves? Consider how medical ways of thinking are affected by the very fact that the community of physicians is professionalized. All professions naturally seek to achieve a certain autonomy, to protect their independence, and to build up specialized bodies of technical expertise (what the medieval guilds called "mysteries") as their private stock in trade. Thus, within any highly professionalized community of practitioners there is a tendency for specific professional roles to be defined narrowly and distinguished sharply from other roles—particularly from those of lay people outside the profession in question. Conversely, we should expect to find practitioners happily accepting very broad definitions of their roles and tolerating extensive overlaps between their own tasks and those of others only in situations where their concerns are organized— if at all—much more loosely than they are in professional organization.

These generalizations hold good not merely for medicine but for all professional enterprises. In these respects there are clear contrasts between physicians and social workers, which parallel those between, for example, steelworkers and fruitpickers. One of the chief by-products of professionalization, as of unionization, is a sharpening and specialization in the demarcation of roles and responsibilities; thus, it should be no surprise that the increasing professionalization of the American medical community during the mid-twentieth century has gone hand in hand with increasingly sharp and specialized definitions of physicians' roles. Nor should it be any surprise that the medical profession has come to organize itself increasingly around the body of technical "mysteries" over which it has some professional monopoly, specifically around applied physiology and biochemistry, or what has come, since 1950, to be known as biomedical science.

In earlier periods, medical practitioners were less organized and also had a much wider vision of their proper roles and responsibilities; they did not hesitate, for instance, to act as personal counselors, community troubleshooters, or even social critics. In these broader roles, they claimed no monopoly of expertise. As personal counselors, they coexisted with the clergy and the lawyers; as community troubleshooters, they played a part alongside the police, the municipality, and all kinds of volunteer workers; and as social critics, they put in their word as citizens having a particular kind of experience, but claimed no greater authority to speak than their fellow citizens. Only their specialized knowledge about the internal physiological workings of the human body set them apart from the rest of the society; it was only this specialized knowledge that could serve to sustain the kind of monopoly which could provide the basis for professional autonomy and self-regulation.

The change in the social organization of medicine and the resulting narrowing of medical responsibilities have had terminological consequences. Earlier, it was customary to distinguish complaints, ailments, and causes that were medical in a narrow sense (i.e., that were open to intervention by the physician alone) from those that were medical in a broader sense (i.e., that called also for personal counseling or even social intervention). More recently, the temptation has been to mark off those conditions that are seen as genuinely medical from others that are, by professional standards, not medical at all. But that narrowing of attention has been question begging.

Philosophically speaking, there is no particular reason to select somatic factors as any more immediately relevant to or causative of human illnesses than all the other kinds of factors and conditions involved. In appropriate contexts, factors and conditions of many different kinds can be spoken of as causing, for example, the businessman's symptoms. Correspondingly, interventions on many levels may provide effective ways of remedying the symptoms and preventing the recurrence of the same complaint. The points at which we might deal with the businessman's condition may be institutional or psychological as much as somatic. Nor is it clear that somatic intervention need be either more effective or more lasting than psychological or social intervention. Surgical treatment of ulcers may lead only to temporary improvement, so long as the patient continues to work under stress; if he changes his job, the ulcers may possibly clear up by themselves without the need for surgery.

Lacking good philosophical reasons to emphasize the somatic conditions of illness, we can recognize more clearly that sociological factors are also involved. If professional physicians today restrict their own roles and limit the permissible range of medical interventions to those about which they have some monopoly of understanding, they will naturally end by concentrating on the physiological and biochemical aspects of human pathology and by developing a correspondingly somatic view of medical causation. Conversely, if they are to develop a broader view of medical causation, they must also widen their ideas about the legitimate loci and modes of intervention, and so about their professional responsibilities: they may accept happily, for instance, the need to counsel patients about their employment, styles of life, personal temperaments, and so on. At times, indeed, they must even be ready, as professionals, to embark on open crusades over matters of public health, industrial organization, and social policy, to the length of staking their reputations—not just their personal reputations, but their reputations as physicians—on the medical importance of those broader issues. Only the lure of that narrow professional autonomy that bases itself on and is nourished by the possession of specialized technical "mysteries" can give the color of a justification to the view that somatic pathologies in themselves are of medical concern, while psychological, social, and political factors have no direct relevance to medicine.

TOWARD A BROADER CONCEPT OF MEDICINE

What are the practical implications of this analysis? The ideal of scientific medicine around which the medical profession has organized itself during the mid-twentieth century, together with the correlative idea of biomedical science on the research front, were historical responses to needs and opportunities that presented themselves in the early years of the century; that much is by now well understood. The reorganization of American medical education stimulated by the Flexner Report, followed by the remarkable improvements in the treatment of infectious diseases associated with the development of antibiotics, are two familiar milestones along this road. But, as is also beginning to be understood, that sequence of historical changes is yielding diminishing returns. Recall the recent California study arguing that cures for the remaining "killer" diseases might add three years to the average expectation of life, whereas changes in people's habits of life could increase it by some eleven years. The needs and opportunities facing the medical profession today are, accordingly, different from those facing physicians in the early years of the century; and these new needs and opportunities also call for new and broader ideas about the character of medical causation. By themselves, however, philosophical arguments can do little to counterbalance the power of professional organization. If it took a revolution in the education and organization of physicians to narrow the attention of physicians to somatic causes, it may well take another revolution in education and organization to broaden those ideas again.

The problems facing medicine, in this respect, are by no means unique. As Hans Jonas's work on responsibility and technology reminds us, they represent only one special illustration of the more general problems associated with the development and application of new technologies. The more technical our lives become, the more dependent we are on the expertise of different professional engineers and the like, the more urgent it is to develop institutional arrangements through which those professional groups can be made answerable to the rest of the community for the social priorities guiding the practical use of their expertise. Without such institutional arrangements, professional autonomy risks turning into professional irresponsibility. Every monopoly dreams, of course, of being permitted to monitor and police its own activities. This was true of the oil trusts at the turn of the century, and it is true of the trade unions today. But once the activities of any monopoly begin to engage the public interest on a large scale—begin, not just to attract public attention, but also to affect the public welfare—this self-monitoring can no longer be enough. It never has worked in the past, and it is unreasonable to suppose that it will work in the future.

At a meeting several years ago, Peter B. Hutt, former general counsel at the Food and Drug Administration, lectured the scientific community on the need to cooperate in the development of institutional arrangements for scientists to exercise their public responsibility in the case of problems like those of recombinant DNA. The scientists pleaded, as eloquently as John D. Rockefeller had seventy-five years before, that they could be trusted to run their own affairs in the public interest, and therefore should be left alone. The medical profession at the present time no doubt feels just the same way. But special pleading is special pleading, whoever engages in it. In the long run, the only questions about the institutional arrangements by which physicians, too, exercise their collective responsibility for the social priorities guiding the practical use of modern medical technologies are how soon they will be set up, and how they can be made to operate in the public interest without appearing needlessly obstructive to the profession.

Pessimistic observers are doubtful whether these new arrangements can be established as quickly or effectively as they need to be, given the entrenched organizational power of the medical profession itself. For sociological and political reasons, they see the current structure of the medical profession, and the methodology of which it has a monopoly and to which it has become accustomed, as having an inertia too great to be changed in less than a generation. Their pessimism is understandable and hard to undermine. One can only reply that, in earlier times, equally powerful interests were in fact obliged to accept a necessary degree of social accountability by the political action of the federal government. One can only hope that, with the increasing development of health maintenance organizations and the like, the tide of opinion among practicing physicians may begin before too long to flow the other way.

How can these changes come about? First, issues in social medicine, public health, personal histories and habits, and even the politics of social reform, must come to be regarded by physicians as having a genuine relevance and significance for medicine equal to, and on an intellectual par with, those of somatic factors. In addition, they must be seen by medical students in training to be so regarded by their professional teachers and role models. Only then shall we find ourselves educating a generation of medical practitioners capable of viewing medical causation with some real philosophical breadth and ready to play their part, as professional physicians, in "promoting health and fighting disease" by intervening in the entire concatenation of relevant factors, conditions, and causes at whatever points will be most efficacious and not merely by manipulating the safe and customary somatic factors.

If we are to broaden our conception of medical practice in this way, it will also be necessary to establish new career ladders and develop new institutions to go with them. State and municipal governments already provide some openings for physicians with special qualifications in public health, factory clinics provide some openings in industrial medicine, and so on. But the powers of the public health authorities are severely limited: school nurses and physicians have more chance to perform inoculations and bandage grazed knees than they do to persuade pupils not to take up smoking, and few factory physicians would be thanked if they tried to intervene directly in the organization of production. Yet, once again, such interventions would not be without precedent. The late-nineteenth century physicians of Barre, Vermont, who saw their patients dying of silicosis as a result of working in dust-filled, unventilated granite cutting shops, did not hesitate to speak up as physicians. Through an active campaign of political action, they were able to shame the state legislature into requiring the installation of proper equipment in the cutting shops to lay the dust and extract it from the air. The embarrassing question to ask today is, Would their present-day successors be as vocal and politically active as they were? Or would they excuse themselves from intervening in the actual operations of the granite shops, claiming that their business was only to treat their patients after they had contracted silicosis, not to help protect them before the event? Looking at the continuing state of affairs in the cotton mills and other industrial plants, one can hardly avoid giving a pessimistic answer here too.

By focusing so narrowly on the somatic aspects of medicine, twentieth-century American physicians have seriously reduced their own effectiveness in the complementary fields of health maintenance and preventive medicine. Philosophically speaking, psychological, social, and political factors have no less right to attention as causes of ill health than do somatic factors. This makes the importance of those neglected enterprises undeniable in theory. But in practice the politics and organization of contemporary medicine in the United States are so deeply committed to and structured by the last half-century's concentration on physiology and biochemistry that those other aspects of medicine are no longer provided for in the average physician's customary habits of thought and action. Professionally and institutionally speaking, therefore, the road back to a more balanced view of medical causation and medical intervention is likely to be long and hard.

Causal Accounts in Medicine:
A Commentary on Stephen Toulmin

H. Tristram Engelhardt, Jr.

What would it mean to have a new understanding of causality in medicine? Presumably, there must be an old understanding with respect to which one forwards revisions, perhaps to take account of better ways of construing causality or of better or more useful ways of viewing the purposes of medicine. Identifying such a new undertaking is difficult because the history of medicine encompasses numerous different past understandings of causality. Moreover, different elements of contemporary medicine employ quite different understandings of causality. Compare, for example, the senses of causality presupposed in psychoanalysis with those in bacteriology, internal medicine, or epidemiology. I will, therefore, select a particular understanding and contrast it with others in order to suggest some ways in which it would be helpful to address current medical concepts of causality and to examine their relation to previous views.

My point of departure will be Stephen Toulmin's helpful essay, "Causation and the Locus of Medical Intervention." I agree with many of Toulmin's views, for example, that a focus on somatic pathologies reflects, in part, the ways in which the community of physicians is organized around views of care and cure, and that causal accounts in medicine function as ways of assigning responsibility in order to signal which of many causal factors are of therapeutic relevance. I agree, as well, that somatic factors should not have the unchallenged claim to priority that they are often accorded; instead, it is important to view broadly the causal factors that are related to the genesis of diseases.

To amplify Toulmin's well-stated positions I will explore and defend the following points: (1) Our current concepts of the role of causality in medicine can be illuminated by an examination of some of the more symptom- or complaint-related approaches of the eighteenth century; (2) The ways in which we view causal connections in medicine today can be better understood if we underscore some of the developments in the nineteenth century that made more somatically oriented accounts appear so attractive; (3) Medicine's treatment of causality functions, as does causation in the law, through deciding what will count as background conditions and what will be treated as causes to be addressed (Hart and Honorè 1959). Where one draws the lines between background conditions and relevant causes is, I will suggest, as much created as discovered by an appeal to the goals of medicine; (4) I will amplify Toulmin's account of why one is often brought to think of causal relations in terms of scientific ideas of causality rather than in terms of everyday or legal views of causation; (5) I will suggest how a reexamination of the goals of medicine, as well as concepts of illness and disease, can suggest ways of analyzing the popular moral imperatives to "treat the patient as a person" and "practice more holistic medicine" with regard to understandings of medical causation. What is interesting about our "new" understandings of causation in medicine is not the accent on psychological, sociological, or political causal factors, but the more instrumentalist view of causation that may lead to the emphasis Toulmin suggests.

I will begin by reexamining Toulmin's example of an individual suffering from an ulcer. The individual is bothered by stomach pains and bleeding, as indicated by his dark stools. One would suspect that he may also be experiencing weakness, faintness, and dizziness, and that he feels chilly and thirsty from his loss of blood. We are told that he is a perfectionist and is subject to stress and frustration. Further, he believes that he must be careful about his diet; evidently, he has a history of intolerance to rich foods. His wife at least partly attributes his problems to the fact that his firm takes advantage of him and that the industrial system takes a heavy toll on executives such as the individual we are considering. In addition, he has a past history of ulcer disease. Though the diagnosis is not certain from the information supplied, I will assume for my discussion that he is suffering from a peptic ulcer.

This individual has a problem that interferes with his ability to accomplish what he wishes to do. He is bothered by stomach pains and, even worse, has just experienced a serious, perhaps potentially life-threatening, episode of internal bleeding. We are interested here in discovering the proper way or ways of talking about the causes of his problems. Toulmin correctly suggests, and very importantly, that we have at least one accepted cause of the symptoms, namely, the ulcer. Stating that the ulcer is the cause of the symptoms may seem to be a trivial causal account. Actually, however, it is a profound move in the history of our approaches to diseases. It provides us with a notion of an underlying pathological process that allows us to collect and view the various signs and symptoms of peptic ulcer disease as manifestations of that underlying lesion. As Horacio Fabrega has argued, this marks an important difference between our biomedical views of diseases and the views of illness of most preliterate societies (1978, pp. 79-107). The idea of an underlying disease process enables us to get behind the symptoms, to assign them a physiological truth value, and to rank them in terms of their physiologically grounded authenticity (Fabrega 1978, pp. 104-05).

This ordering of symptoms and signs has played a central role in the history of our understanding of peptic ulcer disease. Apart from a few extraordinary insights on the part of individuals such as Avicenna, it was not clearly understood until recently that the signs and symptoms of peptic ulcer disease (which we see as the manifestations of an underlying pathological lesion) were, indeed, the result of a gastric or duodenal ulcer. Thus, in the symptom- or complaint-oriented nosologies of François Boisser de Sauvages (1707-1767) and William Cullen (1710-1790), the symptoms of pain and the presentation of rectal bleeding are separated under different major classifications of problems (Sauvages 1769; Cullen 1769). For Sauvages, there are *dolores abdominis*. For Carolus Linnaeus (1707-1778), under *dolorosi* there is *gastrica: ventriculi dolor epigastrii* (1763). William Cullen, in a late edition of his *Nosologia*, lists under *dyspepsia*, which falls under the class *neurosis*, order *adynamiae*, a heading *gastrodynia ulcerosa* (Cullen 1820, p. 95). This occurs under a subdivision of *dyspepsia* labeled *symptomaticae*. The development which led to seeing symptoms as signs of underlying pathological processes reflects the work of patho-anatomists such as Giovanni Morgagni (1682-1771) and his *De sedibus et causis morborum per anatomen indagatis* (1761). There, gastric ulcers receive a description, which was further amplified by Matthew Baillie (1793) and by Jean Cruveilhier in his *Anatomie Pathologique du Corps Humain* (1830-1842).

Such developments have been of immense importance for the manner in which causal accounts are given in medicine. First, signs and symptoms are ordered in terms of underlying pathological mechanisms, so that the search for causes becomes a search for the causes of the underlying pathological processes or lesions. Second, the signs and symptoms no longer have the central role in our attention that they did for Sauvages and Cullen. Third, the sciences of anatomy, physiology, and pathology, which for Sauvages and Cullen were auxiliary sciences, become basic sciences. There is a shift from viewing such sciences as simply helpful in explaining correlations between patients' complaints and other variables, to viewing those sciences as disclosing the true, hidden nature of diseases. That is, they are regarded as basic sciences because they are thought to be able to disclose the relationship between the signs and symptoms of an illness and their underlying basis. This represents a change from the views of physicians such as Sauvages (where the primary goal was to determine correlations of a prognostic and therapeutic sort between signs and symptoms and other variables) to a concern with finding the real causes of disease. Finally this leads to the possibility of a robust explanatory structure capable of distinguishing between the causal mechanisms involved in the pathogenesis of disease (i.e., the mechanisms involved in the evolution of the problems associated with the ulcer—its signs and symptoms) and etiology (the determination of the real cause or causes of the disease entity).

This view suggests that medicine's interest in causes is like the interest of science generally: to portray, apart from any interest in particular goods or values, the causal web of the universe. That is, medicine is cast in the image of an ideal view of the basic sciences, which is moved principally by an interest in knowledge for knowledge's sake. On the basis of knowledge from the basic sciences, medicine then attempts to determine the causal web binding disease entities with the clinician's world, in order to organize or reorganize truthfully the nosological universe. This organization and reorganization of the clinical world in terms of the basic sciences is portrayed in Michel Foucault's *Birth of a Clinic* (1973). However, what he actually portrays is not the birth of a clinic, but, in fact, its subordination to an idealized view of the basic sciences. According to this view, one can come to know the true disease processes underlying the world of the clinician and then discover the causes of those entities.

It has become increasingly apparent that naive hopes of determining the causes of most diseases are not likely to be fulfilled in the near future. Few diseases show the inexorable relationship between cause and effect that rabies displays. Few causes are necessary and sufficient causes of a disease. This is appreciated clearly by Virchow in his *Hundred Years of Pathology* (1895). On the one hand, Virchow argued that the *ens morbi* is a cell or cluster of deranged cells; but on the other hand, he rejected the notion that particular parasites, for example, bacteria, are the *causae morborum*. As he points out by referring to carriers of the diptheria bacillus, the simple presence of the diptheria bacillus is not a sufficient condition for the disease diptheria (1895, p. 38). It is from such considerations that multifactorial views of the etiology of diseases have developed. Though it may be possible to identify certain necessary conditions for a disease, the cluster or clusters of conditions that constitute a sufficient condition have been perceived as ever more complex. Thus, although a disease may have one necessary condition, there may be various patterns of causal variables which are, themselves, insufficient to produce the disease but which can combine with the necessary conditions to produce it.

Faced with a complex constellation of causal factors, few of which are necessary or sufficient, and most of which are unnecessary and insufficient conditions, there is a problem of selecting some for attention. This is the case because, as Toulmin suggests, medicine is far from being a pure science. It is directed instead toward the goal of managing the complaints of patients. To return to Toulmin's example, the man with the peptic ulcer needs help in managing his pain, controlling his bleeding, preventing perforation of his ulcer, avoiding obstruction due to ulcer, and determining whether he has a gastric ulcer (and if so, whether it is cancerous), as well as help in coming to terms with the tensions and vexations that may have expressed themselves in his disease. If one focuses on the patient's complaints and problems, one is likely to rephrase Toulmin's conclusion that medicine should take greater cognizance of the sociological, psychological, and political factors that bear causally upon the development of a peptic ulcer. Instead, a more general point can be sustained, namely, that medicine's concerns with diseases are not primarily etiological. That is, clinical medicine is concerned primarily with managing complaints, not primarily with understanding causes. As a result, as Henrik Wulff has argued, diagnoses are not ends in themselves. Rather, a diagnosis is "a mental resting place for prognostic considerations and therapeutic decisions" which are closely bound to cost-benefit considerations (1976, p. 78). The nosologist's classifications of diseases are, thus, predictive systems in the service of prognosis and therapy rather than primarily causal systems (Wulff 1976, pp. 66-67).

As a consequence, decisions about which causal factors are of interest are based on the costs involved in addressing them and the benefits likely to ensue from giving some center stage. Somatic causal accounts, or psychological, sociological, or political accounts, are given saliency depending upon the cost-benefit consequences of such choices. That is one important reason why Belloc's and Breslow's studies, which suggest that changes in lifestyle would provide much greater increases in longevity than curing all forms of cancer, are so intriguing (Belloc and Breslow 1972; Belloc 1973). They suggest that there may be much cheaper ways (in many senses of cheaper) of coming to terms with the factors that constrain our life expectancy. However, if there were cheaper and more efficacious biological fixes, I am sure that we would choose them in preference. Consider immunization for polio. Even if it were found that polio could be prevented by greatly altering our decadent Western lifestyle, it would probably still be much cheaper and, therefore, preferable simply to immunize.

This can be seen more clearly by reviewing the possible approaches to understanding the etiology of disease. In the case that Toulmin presents (assuming the individual is suffering from a duodenal ulcer), we might begin by seeking a genetic etiology. There appears to be a familial clustering of cases of duodenal ulcers. In addition, the risk of developing a duodenal ulcer is related to blood type: duodenal ulcers are more common in patients with O-type blood than in those who are type A, B, or AB. But although there may be an inclination for peptic ulcers, at present the genetic mechanisms are not sufficiently understood to explain why some individuals' gastroduodenal mucosae fail to withstand the digestive action of the acid-pepsin gastric content, while others do not experience such a failure. Moreover, it is not clear whom such genetic accounts would help.

The search for an etiology may then turn to exploring such factors as hypersecretion of gastric acid, differences in tissue resistance, disturbances in motility, endocrine factors, and other predisposing circumstances. It will be noted, for example, that peptic ulcers are more common when other concurrent diseases are present, such as cystic fibrosis, chronic pulmonary emphysema, chronic pancreatitus, cirrhosis of the liver, or rheumatoid arthritis. However, at best there will be a web of predisposing factors, no one of which is usually a sufficient condition. In fact, though the necessary elements of the pathogenesis of peptic ulcers can be isolated, it is difficult to identify necessary or sufficient etiological factors that bring some individuals to suffer from the disease and others to remain healthy.

One may attempt to account for these differences by an appeal to neuropsychiatric factors. Some psychiatrists have argued that ulcers can develop in individuals with intense parasitic dependent desires; and that individuals who show pseudoindependence, passive dependence, or an expression of their strong oral cravings and demands through pathophysiological symptoms, have an unconscious conflict of dependence versus independence. This conflict, they contend, is causally central to the development of a peptic ulcer (Alexander, French, and Pollack 1968). The etiology of peptic ulcer is thus accounted for in terms of an early oral conflict. Gastric hypersecretors can then be identified as individuals whose oral drives remained ungratified during their infancy because they possessed physiologically insatiable desires (Mirsky 1958). At that point, however, the psychological account of the causation of peptic ulcer collapses into a genetic account or some other nonpsychological explanation, at least for those who are in the possession of such physiologically based insatiable desires.

Depending on which cause or web of causes one selects to be most important for therapeutic reasons, peptic ulcer disease could then be classified as a genetic disease, a psychophysiologic gastrointestinal disorder, or a social disease tied to environmental stresses. It is this instrumentalist character of causal accounts that is central to medicine, as Stephen Toulmin repeatedly suggests. This is a cardinal feature of medicine and should be underscored, for it is a new understanding that enabled medicine simply to discover the causes of diseases. As I have suggested, however, it is a view which has well-established roots—in medicine, as in the law, one chooses those causal factors for attention that are open to useful regard. By choosing where to place its accent of concern, medicine creates a picture of a disease that directs therapy and research. Thus, medical accounts of causation are not simply value-free pictures of the world, but road maps that suggest which approaches are likely to be more successful for the goals and purposes of health care.

Bibliography

Alexander, F., French, T.M., and Pollack, G. 1968. *Psychosomatic Specificity. Volume 1, Experimental Study and Results*. New York: Harper and Row.

Baillie, M. 1793. *Morbid Anatomy of Some of the Most Important Parts of the Human Body*. London.

Belloc, N.B. 1973. "Relationship of Health Practices and Mortality." *Preventive Medicine* 2: 67-81.

Belloc, N.B., and Breslow, L. 1972. "Relationship of Physical Health Status and Health Practices." *Preventive Medicine* 1: 409-21.

Cruveilhier, J. 1830-1842. *Anatomie pathologique du corps humain*. Paris: Bailliere.

Cullen, W. 1769. *Synopsis Nosologiae Methodicae*. Edinburgh: William Creech.

———. 1820. *Nosologia Methodica*. Edinburgh: J. Carfrae.

Fabrega, H. 1978. "Disease Viewed as a Symbolic Category." In *Mental Health: Philosophical Perspectives*, edited by H.T. Engelhardt, Jr. and S.F. Spicker. Boston: D. Reidel Publishing Co.

Foucault, M. 1973. *The Birth of a Clinic: An Archeology of Medical Perception*. New York: Random House.

Hart, H.L.A., and Honorè, A.M. 1959. *Causation in the Law*. London: Oxford University Press.

Linnaeus, C. 1763. *Genera Morborum*. Uppsala: Steinert.

Mirsky, I.A. 1958. "Physiologic, Psychologic and Social Determinants in the Etiology of Duodenal Ulcer." *American Journal of Digestive Diseases* 3: 284-314.

Morgagni, G. 1761. *De sedibus et causis morborum per anatomen indagatis*. Venice.

Sauvages de la Croix, F.B. de. 1768. *Nosologia methodica sistens morborum classes juxta sydenhami mentem et botanicorum ordinem*, 2 volumes. Amsterdam: Fratrum de Tournes.

Toulmin, S.E. 1985. "Causation and the Locus of Medical Intervention," pp. 59-72 in this volume.

Virchow, R. 1895. *Hundert Jahre Allgemeiner Pathologie*. Berlin: C. August Herschwald.

Wulff, H. 1976. *Rational Diagnosis and Treatment*. Oxford: Blackwell Scientific.

Medicine Aimed at the Care of Persons Rather Than What . . . ?

Alasdair MacIntyre

To treat the patient as a *person*—what does that mean? The word has undergone too many transformations in its history and can in different contexts carry with it all too many clusters of conceptual associations for the question to have any easy answer. Originally it was the Latin word *persona*, whose root meaning is that of the mask which the actor wears in the theater, the mask indicating what kind of character the actor is portraying. It came to mean "character" in an extended sense. Cicero, following Panaetius, says that each man has four personae: he is man qua rational animal, man qua this particular individual different from all others, man qua ascribed or endowed social status (inherited wealth or appointment to a military command), and man qua self-chosen sphere of activity (law, philosophy, oratory). Sometimes, indeed, *persona* might even be translated by our word *role*.

The history whereby persons came to be contrasted with the roles that they happen to play is a complex one, and in its course a number of other meanings come into being. The *Oxford English Dictionary* cites "bearer of legal rights" as one meaning of *person*, a meaning in which a corporation can be a person. The meaning of the word may vary from the self-praising of Whitman's line: "What the push of reading could not start, is started by me personally is it not?" to the denigrating "In any case it was just personal" of Fitzgerald's Gatsby.

What then ought we to mean, what can we usefully mean, if we speak of treating patients as persons? I shall in this paper make a suggestion that falls into two parts. First, I shall suggest that the force of speaking in this way characteristically and usefully derives from some contrast that we wish to emphasize. We speak of treating patients as persons rather than in some other way. And one method of stipulating a meaning for the expression "to treat a patient as a person" would be to specify a series of contrasts, so that *as a person* is understood as systematically incompatible with *as a such-and-such* and *as a so-and-so*. But to give a list of such contrasts, although necessary, will not be sufficient; for ruling out a relatively short list of contrasting possibilities would not of itself give any unity to the notion of a person and of treating someone as a person. Hence, my inquiry will move from outlining a series of contrasts to asking in virtue of what it is that one and the same concept is paired with a number of quite different contrast terms.

Each of the three contrasts which I will sketch refers us to a mode of relationship whereby the physician and the patient are likely to systematically misinterpret each other's bearing, behavior, and utterance. Every one of them is the expression of a powerful tendency in our culture which it would be difficult to combat, let alone eliminate, by any simple scheme of reform. I am therefore about to identify difficulties and dangers with which the medical profession will have to live in the foreseeable future, rather than obstacles to be removed. The three types of relationships—which are all too apt to partially define and at the same time to distort the contemporary relationship of the physician to the patient—are that which casts the patient into the role of the client of a bureaucracy, that which casts the physician as an applied scientist and makes of the patient an object of his scientific attention and inquiries, and that which casts the physician in the role of magus or magician. To the examination of each of these I now turn.

MEDICINE AS BUREAUCRACY

Modern medicine is, whether we like it or not, inescapably bureaucratic in its forms. I do not mean by this to refer only to the medicine that is practiced in and through large-scale organizations such as socialized national health services or the health care organizations of large corporations. Even in private practice and in the smaller hospital, the institutionalized setting to a remarkable extent casts the physician in the role of the bureaucrat and the patient in that of the client of a bureaucracy. What are the marks of this particular role relationship? Let me begin with the most superficial aspect.

The patient characteristically has access to the physician only through a prefabricated route in which receptionists, secretaries, and nurses relate to the patient via forms and records. You are, and are invited to become, only and precisely what the form says you are. (You may wish to avoid this by fainting or being knocked down by an automobile just outside a hospital; but emergency rooms too have been remarkably efficient in turning an "emergency" into another routine event.) This has the effect of revealing to the patient the disparity between the anxiety-laden importance which he attaches to the occasion and the unimportance—deriving from its routine character—which the receptionist, secretary, and nurse attach to it. There is nothing in all this that differentiates this occasion from other client-bureaucrat encounters; for example, the visit of an applicant for a loan to a bank officer or the visit of a welfare client to a welfare agency. In all three different types of cases what matters is the routinizing of the case in such a way that it is clear that the bureaucrats are at home in the situation and that the client is not. One way in which this is sometimes accentuated is by well-meant attempts to make the client feel "at home"—the plastic flowers syndrome.

A second characteristic of all bureaucratic relationships is the fact that it is the role that matters and not the individual who fills it. Roles in a bureaucracy are well defined if and only if, when one individual becomes unavailable to fill a role, another can be easily found to take his or her place. Without such substitutability, the continuities characteristic of bureaucratic transactions could not be sustained. If I have a correspondence with General Electric or the IRS, my correspondence is with General Electric or the IRS and not with the particular clerks who draft the letters. The individual clerk or executive is transient; the file is permanent. Files therefore are the essential sustenance of any bureaucracy. When a client visits a bureaucratic office, what matters from the standpoint of the bureaucracy is that he or she sees someone with authority of a certain kind, not some particular individual.

This is also true of modern medicine. Such is the mobility of the modern physician that it is quite possible for a patient to see a different physician on each visit to a clinic; and such is the mobility of the modern patient that a particular instance of a disease or a disorder often enough travels from physician to physician. It is the files—and often only the files—which provide permanence and stability.

What the patient therefore encounters in his or her search for treatment is not so much an individual or even a set of individuals as a form of organization: a ward, a clinic, a hospital, a surgical team. Which particular surgeon operates may be a matter of chance, and the norms of care in a ward will affect the patient's experience far more than the particular nurses who happen to be on duty. This runs counter to the individualistic way in which we have all been trained to think of the doctor-patient relationship. It is notable that when accusations of "ghost surgery" have been made, what has been thought to be wrong has been the violation of a contractual relationship between the individual surgeon, the attending physician, and the individual patient. But this conception of a contract between individuals is now almost entirely legal; it is nothing but the ghost of a largely vanished moral conception which presupposed a stable, long-term relationship between individual patient and individual physician in the context of a particular local community. That relationship was such that particular transactions between doctor and patient had a background in the personal knowledge of each by each, a background which is necessarily missing in the bureaucratic context of modern medicine. Thus, the point is not just that modern medicine is often impersonal in a characteristically bureaucratic way; it is that this impersonality coexists with a quite different individualistic way of thinking about the doctor-patient reality. As a result, the patient experiences not only the impersonality, but also a continuously recurring divorce between expectation and reality. This is perhaps why the appropriate word to express the attitude of many patients to doctors is *disappointment*, a disappointment grounded less in bad diagnosis or failures of treatment than in the absence of an anticipated but necessarily unavailable form of human relationship.

The impersonality of bureaucracy, it ought to be emphasized, is a highly specific form of impersonality with three salient characteristics. The first is the way in which the clients of a bureaucracy are forced into attitudes of dependency. This dependency does not derive from the fact that the client always approaches the bureaucracy with certain needs; it is much more a function of the way in which the bureaucracy preserves and asserts its right to tell the client what his or her needs are. This characteristic is intimately bound up with the forms of self-justification which the members of a bureaucracy deploy toward both the outside world and each other. It is because, and insofar as, a bureaucracy is or seems to be the possessor of skills, information, and expertise that it is able to warrant the claims that it makes both to its clients and to the public at large. It is because, and insofar as, it is able to acquire a monopoly of skills, information, and expertise within a certain area that a bureaucracy is able to make itself both privileged and indispensable, the ideal state to which all bureaucracies aspire. This aspiration for monopolistic privilege is part of the process not only of bureaucratization, but also of professionalization. There are certainly ways in which the membership of a profession and the service of a bureaucracy can be in tension or conflict, but there are also ways in which the two statuses can be mutually reinforcing.

The client, therefore, finds himself confronted by a situation in which the bureaucrat asserts a right not only to identify the solution of the client's problem or to declare that the problem is insoluble, but also a prior right to say what the client's problem is, or even to deny that the client has a problem. The client's right to "answer back" is severely restricted and is often treated as impertinent in both senses of that word. This particular way of reducing the client to dependence is highly characteristic of modern medicine. It is reinforced by the kind of passivity peculiar to the sick role, as analyzed by Parsons (1975) and others. There is interesting empirical evidence that patients who are reluctant or unable to play the part of a patient as that part is conceived by doctors and nurses are likely to be classified as maladjusted and may be discharged from a hospital sooner than those who know how to act the part in the required way (De Longe 1963).

There are other bureaucratic devices which produce client dependency. An important one is making the client wait in line. A central characteristic of modern patient experience is that of waiting for unpredictable amounts of time—waiting to see the nurse, waiting to be examined by the physician, waiting for the results of the blood test or the x-ray. Modern medicine almost always treats the time of physicians and surgeons as extremely valuable (and rightly so), and the time of patients as extremely valueless. In so doing, it devalues the patient as well as the patient's time, and in this it is no different from social welfare and unemployment agencies. The end result is, once again, increased client dependency.

A second relevant characteristic of bureaucracies is the way in which they deal with error. Bureaucracies tend to prohibit, so far as possible, any admission of error *to* the client, and thus give the appearance of trying to assume a pose of infallibility in their relations to the external world. Consequently, within the bureaucratic organization there will be widely recognized informal rules which induce and sometimes enforce cooperation in removing the appearance of error. These informal rules—they have to be informal, for the promulgation of formal rules would defeat the purpose of those rules—in turn produce a limited measure of cooperation in removing the appearance of error within the organization. The result is a climate in which the open acknowledgment of error is penalized and no one keeps systematic records of errors. Here again, modern medicine is no different from other modern bureaucracies: the inability of the medical profession to acknowledge and confront the facts of medical error is one more characteristic bureaucratic inability (imagine the impossibility of a sign in a room where patients are waiting which announces, "About three-fifths of you will benefit from being here and 5 percent may suffer positive harm").

The third relevant characteristic of bureaucracy is face-saving; this is clearly related to the inability to admit error but needs to be distinguished from it. The classical account was given by Tom Burns in his study of managers in a firm that was experiencing rapid technological change. Managers were able to give a clear and well-organized account of the rule-governed progress of their activities until just prior to the present phase of those activities, and an equally clear and well-organized account of how their work would proceed in the future; however, they treated the present as an interlude of improvised coping with some emergency or abnormal situation. Burns's finding suggests the thesis that all organizations have a picture of their own normal working, which they project onto their past and their future, but which the members are aware is only very imperfectly instantiated in the present. There is, that is to say, a sharp contrast between the ostensible working by rules and routines and the actual series of improvisations by which the appearance of so working is maintained. Thus, the maintaining of bureaucratic appearances, the saving of institutional face, is the counterpart of coping with the unpredicted which keeps invading even the best-run organizations. From the client's point of view, what matters is the apparent inability of bureaucracy to admit this constant recommitment to the task of deceiving both themselves and their clients about the way they operate. Hence, strict truthfulness is a virtue that is necessarily disruptive of bureaucratic forms, and naively truthful persons can expect to find their transactions with bureaucracies peculiarly disturbing.

It is crucial to emphasize that this account of bureaucracy does not point to any easy moral conclusions. Bureaucratic modes of relationship are unavoidable facts of contemporary social life. Without bureaucracies a large number of essential services, including health care, could not be delivered to mass populations. To some extent the physician is compelled to play the role of bureaucrat and the patient that of client; the problems can be realistically formulated only after this has been acknowledged. Nonetheless, it is clear that insofar as the physician treats the patient as a bureaucratic client, he or she fails to treat the patient as a person. Thus, one dimension of our initial problem is revealed.

The roots of the problem lie in a characteristic of bureaucracies which has already been noted, but which now needs to be given added emphasis. There is a crucial discrepancy between the client's definition of his or her own good and needs and the bureaucracy's definition of the client's good and needs. This discrepancy is mirrored in the difference between the patient's self-defined good and the physician's definition of the patient's good. The patient wants to recover his health in such a way that he recognizes himself as healthy; the physician's goal is to restore the patient's health by treating a set of identifiable diseases or disorders. These two definitions of the patient's good are not extensionally equivalent. Hence, the recurring experiences of the patient seeking medical care who is told that he is perfectly healthy, and of the patient who is certain that he is perfectly healthy being told that there is something very wrong. In one sense the physician is right far more often than the patient. But in another sense, in the last analysis, only the patient has the right to give the verdict. The physician's good has to be defined in terms of the patient's good and not vice versa. Although the patient is not free to define his good qua health as he wishes, nonetheless the patient's health must be that which is defined as health by the patient. Health and illness are necessarily and unalterably prescientific concepts of everyday life. Thus, the physician's scientific competence does not entail, quite apart from other considerations, the physician's medical competence, which is competence in promoting the patient's self-defined good. There is always potential and often actual conflict between the duty of a physician and the role of a bureaucrat. A key part of the life of a modern physician who is necessarily a bureaucratic physician consists in negotiating a way through that conflict.

THE PHYSICIAN AS AN APPLIED SCIENTIST

I turn now to a second role that partially defines the modern physician-patient relationship. This role is rooted not so much in the general history of our culture as is the role of the bureaucrat, but much more in the specific history of twentieth-century medicine. For the victories of medicine in the last sixty years have largely been the victories of applied science. It is no accident that the specializations of medicine have tended to correspond to the subdivisions of the natural sciences, and that the medical division of labor has been one more example of the scientific division of labor. It is because of the application of the sciences that we in America do not now, as we did in 1900, most often die of major infectious conditions, but instead live long enough to die of heart disease, stroke, and cancer.

Part of our inheritance from this period, in which successful medicine was successful applied science, is a view of the patient as essentially either an object for or an exemplification of the results of scientific research. Viewed thus, the patient is no longer envisaged as a whole person, but only as a body; and the body itself is envisaged as a collection of parts and subsystems, each of which may fruitfully be studied in isolation from the rest. According to this view of medicine, the physician reenacts with the parts of a patient's body what the scientist had first achieved on the laboratory bench, and it follows that the specific complaints uttered by the patient and the care of the patient are not really part of the genuine practice of medicine at all. The total subordination of the nurse to the physician has the same rationale as the total subordination of the laboratory technician to the physiologist or biochemist. The physician's belief in the incompetence of the patient with regard to his or her own condition has the same rationale as the incompetence of rats with regard to psychology.

One effect of this focus of attention is to render several aspects of the human being invisible to the physician. For to view the human being as an assemblage of bodily parts and processes is to deprive the patient qua patient of every moral as well as every social dimension. This ensures that a variety of types of cause and effect of medically important conditions are obscured from view, types of cause and effect which it is less and less easy to ignore as medical attention moves from the infectious conditions to the major chronic conditions. Stress and anxiety, conditions experienced in the family and the workplace, the quality of care, the patient's hopes, fears, and expectations—factors which stubbornly resist operational definiton because of their intentional character—become crucial both to explanation and to therapy. It becomes clear that we are at a very primitive stage in constructing medical narratives. For we have one story to tell which is a segment of the patient's biography: it is the patient who is angry or bereaved or out of work, who mourns or drinks or takes to his bed, who worries too much about his work, who hates the nurse or the surgeon. And we have another story to tell which seems not to be about the patient at all, but only about his blood pressure and cholesterol level, about damaged muscles or emphysematous lungs. The true medical narrative must be able to unify those two stories, and we know how to do this only in the most primitive way. This inability does not derive from any inadequacy peculiar to the theory or the practice of medicine; it derives from the way in which our culture, in thinking about human beings, oscillates between two unsatisfactory metaphysical alternatives: an inadequate materialism and an equally inadequate dualism. Sometimes we behave like the heirs of Descartes, at others like those of La Mettrie. Because of this oscillation we tend to revert to a simple but false and distorting reductionist view of both the nature of science and the nature of the patient. Thus, there is always a tension between the kind of focus of attention which a physician qua physician owes to his patients as part of his duty toward them and the focus of attention which that same physician qua scientific researcher will be apt to direct toward the bodies of these same patients. Not every physician is a scientific researcher; nonetheless, the dilemmas arising from this necessarily double vision are, in the long run, as important to the profession as a whole, as are the conflicts between the role of physician and the role of bureaucrat.

THE PHYSICIAN AS MAGUS

The roles of bureaucrat and client are thrust upon the physician and the patient by the general social and economic order of modernity;

the role of "object of scientific research" is thrust upon the patient by a certain kind of physician. I turn now to a role that the patient projects onto the physician in such a way that it scarcely matters that the physician himself would never be likely to employ it. The role in question is that of the magus, of the magician or wizard. When I assert that the contemporary patient is all too apt to treat the physician as a magus, I intend this as no vague simile, but in a very precise way. I must therefore, even if briefly, say what I mean by magic and indicate the conditions in which it flourishes.

There are two ways of understanding magic which I must immediately reject. One assimilates it to science, the other to religion. In the first view, magical practices are ineffective attempts to control natural and social phenomena by people whose culture is not sufficiently advanced to provide them with the instruments of control which derive from the natural sciences. This view of magic, as a kind of primitive and unsuccessful science, embodies two distinct mistakes. The first is the supposition that magic and science are rival attempts to explain the same phenomena; in fact, magic and science direct their attention to quite different classes of phenomena. The bacteriologist or the virologist explains why this person (or any person similarly circumstanced) contracted (or would have contracted) this infection; the practitioner of witchcraft or magic explains why this particular person (and no one else) contracted the infection soon after, for example, insulting someone. To the question: "Why did Jones develop measles immediately after his quarrel with Smith?", natural science—as some modern defenders of African witchcraft like to point out—has no answer.

The second mistake of those who take magic to be would-be science is the failure to recognize the difference between science's claim to knowledge and magic's claim to power. For the magician, knowledge is only a means to the end of power, and more particularly, power which remains the property of the magician. Hence, if one came to believe in the claim of the natural sciences, the appropriate next step would be to learn, to acquire a scientific education; by contrast, if one comes to believe in the claims of magic, the appropriate next step is to find and employ, if one can, a magician.

The confusion between magic and religion is of a different kind. The temptation to assimilate magic to religion arises from the fact that both types of practice seem to claim to put us in touch with sources of supernatural power. One crucial difference is that theistic religion at least claims to put us in the hands of a power which we cannot and must not try to control—"Nevertheless not my will but thine" is the paradigmatic theistic prayer—whereas magic claims to put us in touch with a power which the magician controls and is able to summon at will by formula or ritual. A second difference between magic and theistic religion is that the salvation offered by theistic religion carries no guarantee of preservation from suffering, pain, or death. We can be blessed by God, we can be as good as Job, and yet suffer the worst of brutalities and indignities. Magic, by contrast, promises us power that is effective now against disease, bad harvests, and all the afflictions of our fragile and vulnerable existence; it is an attempt to make us invulnerable. Where magic is talismanic, theistic religion is sacramental.

The eighteenth-century Enlightenment saw both religion and magic, if it ever distinguished them, as forms of superstition that would gradually be eliminated with the progress of science and rational education. It thus failed to foresee two striking and closely linked developments in twentieth-century America. One is the ability of advanced science and technology to coexist with the most blatant forms of superstition; in our own culture the state of California is notable both as a home of science and science-based industry and as a refuge for every kind of magical cult. It is in university towns that astrology tends to flourish. There are at least modest grounds for the hypothesis that in the absence of a general religious culture, science and superstition are symbiotic rather than mutually hostile. A second development is the magical understanding of science itself. The emphasis by would-be spokesmen for science on science as a means of power and control, coupled with a lack of understanding by much of the population of the fallibility at the heart of science, can easily suggest that a good deal of science is a kind of magic. Of no part of science is this more often true than it is of medical science.

Recall the distinctive characteristics of the magus: the ability to understand and explain why I personally have been the victim of this terrible disaster, and the possession of the power to make me better and also to make me invulnerable and immortal. The only problem is how to find the magus and offer an adequate reward for using that power for my magical benefit! This is how many people in our culture think of and act toward the physician and the medical scientist. They look to medicine not merely for the relief of this pain or the alleviation of this disaster, but for something that will prevent them from growing old. They want to remain young and young looking. They want death fended off indefinitely and they do not want one set of diseases and disorders cured merely so that they can later suffer and die from some other set of diseases and disorders. They want *everything* cured: cancer, heart disease, lung disease, kidney disease, *any* disease. They look for and believe in miracle drugs. They do indeed want to become invulnerable and immortal. They project onto the physician the powers of and the role of the magician.

The natural sequel to this attitude is disillusionment, a disillusionment that may take two different forms. One is simple hostility to physicians, a hostility which strengthens that climate in which the will to bring malpractice suits is fostered. The other is the replacement of an irrational faith in orthodox medicine by an irrational faith in some unorthodox mode of practice or nostrum: homeopathy, Laetrile therapy, or whatever. Although the role of magician is projected onto rather than assumed by the physician, it is, nonetheless, the physician and the entire practice and profession of medicine which are apt to suffer from this particular confusion of roles. The belief in magic is, if I am right, deeply rooted in our culture and in the particular kinds of anxieties and dissatisfactions which a secular, rootless mode of life engenders. Thus, here again, there are conflicts and tensions to be negotiated.

TREATING PATIENTS AS PERSONS

If the physician and patient are bound to misinterpret each other, if they allow their transactions to be defined in terms of the relationships between the bureaucrat and client, between the scientific researcher and the object of his inquiries, or between the magus and his would-be disciple, how ought the physician to envisage and treat the patient? What should be the positive content of the phrase "to treat the patient as a *person*"? We need to avoid two opposite mistakes at this point.

The first mistake would be easy to fall into. If physician and patient are pressured by the general culture into miscasting each other into a variety of roles, ought not each instead ask what the other is *really* like as he is in himself, apart from all roles? The notion that the true self is a self that exists apart from the roles it happens to play and the position it happens to occupy is an idea that has long endured. But it is a false conception and a particularly dangerous one when applied by physicians to patients. Why is it false? And why is it dangerous?

It is false because, apart from all role-defined relationships, a human being is not truly an individual, but is emptied of human substance. We are what we are in virtue of our relationships, and we value what we do because of the goods discovered in and through the activities which constitute these relationships. I pursue my good qua father or qua son, my good qua farmer or qua teacher of philosophy, my good qua gardener or ballplayer. And there is of course my good qua me, that peculiar blend of all those role-defined goods which constitutes the *telos* of my particular life. But abstract me from all my roles and what is left is necessarily a life without a *telos*, without form, a set of unordered needs and wants with nothing to bind them into a whole. Thus, the patient, as he or she is, is the patient defined by and acting within those roles which constitute his or her family and home life, his or her life in the local and in the larger community. Hence, to approach the patient as he or she is must be to approach the patient in the context of all these activities and all these relationships. This is why it is false for the physician to think of the patient's having a reality apart from these roles. But why is it dangerous to do so?

The answer is that serious illness is one of a series of conditions— for example, unemployment, vagrancy, madness and going on vacation—in which people are removed from the network of role relationships and activities which constitute their lives so that they actually become, to some extent, an impoverished shadow of their true everyday self. The patient, like the vagrant or the man for whom a vacation is the suffering of empty leisure, is transformed to some degree into that set of unordered needs and wants without a guiding *telos* which at first seemed a conceptual mistake rather than a true image of a human being. Actually, it turns out to be a true image, but only of a human being suffering from grave deprivation and distortion. What I am characterizing is of course an extreme state toward which particular patients or the unemployed or vagrants may only have moved in a limited way. Nonetheless, it is this aspect of a patient's life which leads to many of the familiar phenomena of the "sick role" (Levine and Kozloff 1978). And it is this which makes it so easy for the physician to miscast and misconceive the patient either by his own unrecognized role-governed perception of the patient, or by his failure to recognize the patient's own misperception of himself.

The other mistake, a counterpart to the first, is to suppose that in order to respect the patient as a person we have to respect his or her individual autonomy. From what I said earlier about the false roles into which physician and patient cast each other, we can see that the physician must take three essential precautions in order to negotiate successfully the difficulties of being a bureaucrat, a scientific researcher, and a supposed magus. First, the patient must be supplied with what is in substance (although not in technical vocabulary or scientific depth) the same information—including the same weighing of probabilities and doubts—that the physician possesses. Second, the patient must make all the key decisions which concern his or her good within certain broad limits; the patient's good must remain self-defined. Third, the patient should be made aware of all the possibilities of medical error present in his or her situation. The systematic implementation of this third step would effectively destroy the fantasy of the physician as magus; the systematic implementation of the first two would provide at least partially effective counterweights to the tendencies to make the patient into a bureaucrat's client or a mere object of scientific inquiry.

But there is, however, a crucial objection, one that is often argued within the medical profession, to making any of these precautions routine parts of medical practice and procedure; namely, that the patient, abstracted and isolated from his everyday roles and activity, would not be liberated and rendered autonomous by these measures. Instead, it is argued, the patient would be overwhelmed and rendered incapable of any genuinely rational or autonomous response by being made, in effect, the "victim" of all this information, doubt, and hesitancy, just when there is the greatest need for immediate and forthright decision. And this objection clearly has great force so long as it is the characteristically abstracted and isolated patient of the "sick role" with whom we are dealing. If there is an answer to this powerful objection, it is to be found by reconsidering the nature of autonomy and rationality.

Autonomy is not, as Kant thought, a property of every rational agent. It is an achievement and a social achievement, as is rationality itself. It is in and through our network of relationships that we achieve or fail to achieve rational control of our lives. We are sustained, corrected, and educated by our family ties, our work relationships, and our friendships. It is in and through a variety of dialogues and practical transactions that decisions are tested and criticized, new ideas formulated, older beliefs reformulated. It is the habit of our culture to abstract the final products of the decision-making process which are uttered in an individual voice—the particular decision, argument, or expression of belief—from the social relationship and processes which led to their production. Hence, if we are to look for autonomy and rationality, we should seek them not in individuals abstracted and isolated from their social roles and relationships, but in individuals at home in those roles and relationships. The moral for medical practice is clear, even if in present circumstances utopian: to treat the patient as a person in any substantial sense we must refuse to direct our medicine toward individuals abstracted from their social roles and relationships. The home and the workplace have to become the locus of medical practice; the family and the working group—and not the individual apart from his or her ties—must become the objects of medical attention. To call this proposal utopian is to draw attention to the difficulties that would confront any attempt to transform medical practice in this direction. But the arguments elsewhere in this paper show us what harms and dangers, what misunderstanding and mistreatment, we shall perpetuate if we fail to transform it.

Bibliography

De Longe, W. 1963. "Patient Role Conflict and Reactions to Hospitalization." *Journal of Health and Human Behavior* 4: 113-18.

Levine, S., and Kozloff, M.A. 1978. "The Sick Role: Assessment and Overview." *American Review of Sociology* 4: 317-43.

Parsons, T. 1975. "The Sick Role and the Role of the Physician Reconsidered." *Milbank Memorial Fund Quarterly* 53: 257-78.

Philosophical Groundings for Treating the Patient as a Person: A Commentary on Alasdair MacIntyre

Edmund D. Pellegrino

> ... and you doctors are the champions, the strategists, in the struggle of the individual life against the law of life.
>
> —Paul Valéry

Professor MacIntyre's essay puts squarely before us what may be the most crucial question in this conference. "To treat the patient as a *person*—what does that mean?" he asks (1985, p. 83). The question is crucial because the way we answer uncovers our philosophy of medicine and also grounds our concept of medical morality, telling us what patients may expect and what physicians must provide in the central act of medicine, the relationship between one person— a professed healer—and another person in need of healing.

There is much anxiety today among patients and physicians because of the uncertain state of the answer to this crucial question. Patients fear a loss of personal identity in the complexities of modern medical care; physicians become confused about the potential conflict between curing and caring. Both are tempted to extremes. Patients may yield either to a total dependence that eschews personal decision and invites paternalism, or to total independence and self-healing. Physicians may incline either to an ethos of clinical science that excludes everything not subject to specific cure, or to a vague medical holism that makes medicine the salvation of all human ills.

The extremes of these antinomies are dangerous to the central concern of the medical encounter—a right and good healing action for a particular patient in a particular set of clinical and life circumstances. Patients and physicians urgently need some philosophically grounded resolution of the dilemmas and tensions induced by uncertainty about the critical aspect of their relationships (Pellegrino 1979).

Professor MacIntyre gives a two-part answer to his question: he tells what treating the patient as a person does not mean and then he defines its positive content.

First, he tells us what he does not mean by showing how personhood is violated if the physician succumbs totally to three predominant characteristics of modern medicine and becomes merely a scientist, bureaucrat, or magus. Each distorts and depersonalizes the healing relationship in a specific way. With this formulation I fully agree. I agree, too, that the tendencies MacIntyre ascribes to contemporary medical care will not disappear. Our task must be to find ways, despite these tendencies, to preserve the personal integrity of the patient.

I disagree, however, with the second part of MacIntyre's argument— his prescription for the positive content of treating the patient as a person. I disagree on two counts: first, with his recommendation that the dilemmas can be resolved by making the family and the workplace the locus of care, and more particularly, with the ontology of person that underlies his positive recommendations. For ultimately it is what we think a person is that determines how he should be treated when he is ill.

My disagreement focuses on the one-sidedness of MacIntyre's theoretical and practical formulation. Fleeing from the errors of an atomistic conception of personhood, MacIntyre falls into the opposite error of social determinism. The virtue of MacIntyre's argument rests in his emphasis on the importance of life role in making persons ill and making them well; its defect lies in his abnegation of the needs of the person as a unique being distinct from the roles he occupies. MacIntyre ignores the complementarity of individual and social existences. These complimentarities are essential to our definition as persons; to lose one or the other is to lose the fullness of human personhood.

Each person lives and dies, is ill or well, in a simultaneity of isolation and relationships. Simone Weil gave voice to our isolation as persons when she said, "Every being cries out to be read differently." Charles Péguy, on the other hand, recognized how our existence is linked to our social milieu when he said, "When a man dies, he dies not just of the disease he has; he dies of his whole life."

MacIntyre argues that medicine has erred seriously in isolating the person as patient from his social context, from the roles he plays in the family, at work, in society. He goes further and avers that these roles and relationships define the person and that beyond them there is no identity. In place of the atomistic, autonomous conceptions of personhood, MacIntyre would install a socially determined identity. "We are what we are in virtue of our relationships, and we value what we do because of the goods discovered in and through the activities which constitute these relationships" (p. 93). He even grounds all the essential features of personhood, and any autonomy and rationality the person may possess, in a "network of role relationships" (p. 94). The person, in MacIntyre's view, is coterminous with his role relationships and really has no existence outside the context of those relationships.

If we accept MacIntyre's ontology of personhood, then the positive content of treating the patient as a person must conform closely to the context of social and role relationships. Disease itself becomes a manifestation of distortions in role relationships because the whole being of the person is imbedded in those relationships. Healing must primarily reverse or ameliorate disturbed role relationships and the proper locus for medicine is, indeed, squarely in the nexus of the malfunctioning relationships that have produced the disease.

We can acknowledge the contribution to illness of disturbances in role relationships and their reversal in cure without accepting MacIntyre's ontology of person as a socially determined entity. MacIntyre could have made his point without overshooting the mark so drastically. He has chosen, however, to justify his prescriptive notions by a firm ontological stance. His theory of healing must in consequence be so one-sided. It becomes necessary, therefore, to propose an alternative conception of personhood that I believe is more consistent with the realities of illness and healing.

The history of attempts to derive an ontology of personhood goes back at least to Boethius (475-524). These attempts continue in contemporary philosophy and psychology, especially those of the phenomenologic and existentialist persuasions. With no pretense to doing justice to that history, I wish to emphasize two aspects of the ontology of personhood most pertinent to the positive content of what it means to treat the patient as a person.

The first aspect is our understanding of the concept of a person. I do not think anything written since can improve on Boethius's definition of a person as "an individual substance of a rational nature." The person is a unit member of a species and therefore an individual entity distinct from other unit members of that species. But to be an individual is not to be a person. It is in the possession of rationality as part of his nature that man becomes a person, an individual distinct from other individuals. Even if this rationality cannot always be expressed—in the fetus, in infancy, in sleep, or in coma—it is the capability of rationality as an intrinsic part of his or her nature that makes each man and woman a person. That rationality inheres in a substratum, a continuous, historical being, that underlies thought and action and to which thought and action can be attributed.

Rationality I construe in the usual sense of the capability of forming ideas, making judgments, and arriving at conclusions. Most crucial to this discussion is the reflexive nature of human rationality, the capacity to think about one's thoughts, to examine them critically, to see alternatives and make choices among competing value systems, and thus to act morally. This capability is exercised on all aspects of presenting reality, one's own thoughts, relationships with others, the world, and God. It demands freedom to make choices since the choices must be our own. Freedom is therefore the first obligation owed to persons qua persons. Without freedom, personhood cannot come into full being.

In the second sense, somewhat more phenomenologically, we can construe personhood as the product of this rational capability of individual substances. That product is the configuration of rational choices we have made as a result of the creative interaction between our internal demands, desires, and strivings and those of the external world. What we accept and what we reject in that interaction—the sum total of those choices—defines us as *this* person, not just another instance of this species. No two persons make precisely the same choices and so our choices define us as unique beings, as *this person*, not the universal person.

An essential element in this aspect of personhood is a selective interaction with other persons who constitute our social relationships and our roles. But this cannot be the sole definition of our personhood because we accept some things and reject others in our relationships with others. There is a substratum, distinct from these relationships, that makes choices and can transcend the demands of roles, relationships, and culture. That substratum is never wholly definable and never would be, even if we could enumerate all our roles and relationships and any other observable characteristics. It is the substratum beyond these accidentals to which we attribute the moral responsibility of persons. Morality does not exist for other animal species since they do not perceive right and wrong or have the capacity to make rational choices between them.

These two facets of personhood—its rational nature and its expression in the personal identity that results from use of that rationality—are central to any definition of the positive content of treating the patient as a person. To see this more clearly, we must first see how the fact of illness may alter these aspects of personhood.

Illness and other physical impairments cannot alter the ontological nature of human personhood because that resides in a capability and not in its actual expression. Illness is, however, a serious assault on the actual expression of personhood, on the freedom to make choices, to fashion a personal identity, and to reshape that identity in response to our changing life experiences. When he senses himself as ill, the patient perceives a transformation in his personal existential status. He has become *Homo patiens*, a man bearing a burden of pain, anxiety, or disability. He is marked off from the universe of those who are healthy. He recognizes that he is still a person but a person in a partially impaired state. A patient is a member of a subset of humanity characterized by the loss of crucial freedoms—those we normally associate with being fully persons.

Illness places physical and emotional impediments on our choices. We can no longer use the body for transbodily purposes as a means to our self-defined ends. Instead, it takes center stage as the focus of our concerns and demands to be served rather than serving. In the case of emotional illnesses the psyche becomes an impediment in the same way.

More important are the impediments illness imposes on the exercise of the actual capacity for rational choice. The sick person lacks the knowledge to decide what to do to heal himself. He also lacks the skill to use what knowledge he does have, or gains, about his illness. He must seek out others and he is dependent on that other person who controls what information he receives. Even to begin to make his own choices, the sick person must expose his vulnerability to another who might manipulate or even deceive him in his choice.

Finally, illness challenges the product of our past exercise of rational choice—the self-image we have constructed of ourselves. That image is carefully constructed of choices and compromises, but on the whole it is in dynamic equilibrium with our existential state. That equilibrium is seriously perturbed by the eruption of illness into our lives. Illness forces the reshaping of a new equilibrium through a new set of decisions often having unwelcome alternatives. To become a diabetic, a cardiac, or a patient with cancer awaiting death demands the most fundamental reconstruction of personal identity.

That reconstruction is managed, so to speak, by the "I," the historical continuing entity that persists beneath all changes, past and future. It is the urgency and specificity of the assault of illness on the patient's freedom to become a person that generates the cry for help, the cry to be healed and made whole again. The patient wants to be free again to make his own choices, define his own ends and choose the kind of life he wishes to live.

Social relationships no doubt condition the reconstruction of personal identity in illness, but they are not the whole ground of identity. The "I" interacts with the other, but it is out of the interaction that a new equilibrium with the life situation emerges. Ultimately the experience of illness is not fully communicable to others; hence its challenges are lonely ones. That experience may dictate opening up, or closing off, new roles and relationships, but always there is a choice to be made by the unchanging substratum of decision making—the person who is ill.

This concept of personhood is more concretely expressed in the expectations the sick person holds of those who presume to heal him. I can define the positive content of what it means to treat the patient as a person by reviewing those expectations as I have heard them repeatedly expressed in my years as a clinician. I can paraphrase those expectations in an extended cry for help:

Listen to me—hear what I mean by being ill; listen to what illness is doing to *me*, to my conception of life, to the kind of person I am and want to be, a person of this age, this family, this set of hopes, these frustrations, this history. I am not the universal patient. I am *this* patient. My experience of illness is unique for me; you can't heal me unless you understand my illness and only I can tell you about my unique experience of it.

Please understand that I am impaired and wounded in my person and therefore vulnerable before your knowledge and skill which I need to make me whole. To heal me you must also help me repair my personhood, regain those freedoms of self-determination I have lost through illness. Don't take advantage of my vulnerability to humiliate me or advance your own interests, to treat me as an object, a disease, a case; don't diminish my already diminished person even further.

Our relationship is one of inequality in which you, the healer, have all the power. Please reduce that inequality by helping me to know what is wrong, how serious it is, what you plan to do, what alternatives I have. I want to know whether your treatment is worthwhile for *me*. Even if it is worthwhile for others it may not suit my version of what is good in life.

Please try to understand the uniqueness of the assault this illness makes on this person, on me. Have compassion; feel something of my distress as you undertake to diagnose, treat, and prognosticate. Your general rules, your techniques, must be operative in my unique personal experiences of life and illness.

The positive content of treating the patient as a person consists in heeding these pleas of the one who is ill. It means that the physician, nurse, psychologist—all who profess healing—must repair to the extent possible those impairments to the expression of personhood that disease entails. Obviously, the pathology of body and psyche must be reversed by the most competent and effective technical measures. But all must be done so as to enhance also the person's capability to redefine his or her own identity as a self-determining being.

The patient as person is, therefore, owed the restoration of certain freedoms since freedom is the first condition of the expression of personhood. Truth must be told, facts disclosed, and alternatives set forth fairly and clearly. Consent must not be manipulated; the patient must not be humiliated by condescension, however benign. We must ask what the patient thinks is wrong, what the patient wants to achieve in life, what he deems important, and what treatment objective he deems worthwhile.

These are some of the things that make up the positive content of treating the patient as a person. They become moral obligations that bind all who profess to heal. Healing means to make whole and to repair insofar as possible what illness does to this person. This is the promise inherent in the act of profession, and it is made every time a health professional presumes to undertake treatment of another person.

The scientific, bureaucratic, and magical characteristics of contemporary medicine make the fulfillment of these obligations more difficult than ever. They cannot, however, absolve the professions from meeting them. Indeed, with a proper ontology of personhood and of the impairments illness imposes on its expression, the person of the patient need not be lost even amid the complexities of modern medicine.

In sum, then, MacIntyre's analysis of the threats to treatment of the patient as a person is correct. His remedy—relocating medicine in the family and workplace—has merit as an antidote to the isolation of the patient's treatment from his social matrices. It is an incomplete solution because it ignores the uniqueness of the experience of illness, of the person's role as determinant of his own healing, as well as the complementarity of isolation and relation in all human existence. This can be as dangerous as the overemphasis on isolation and autonomy which MacIntyre deplores. What is primarily at fault is MacIntyre's unbalanced concept of personhood as determined solely by social and role relationships. I have proposed a more balanced concept that permits attention to both the social and the individual aspects of illness and healing. It is on this concept that the positive content of the admonition to treat the patient as a person must be built.

Bibliography

MacIntyre, A. 1985. "Medicine Aimed at the Care of Persons Rather Than What ... ?", pp. 83-96 in this volume.

Matthews, J., ed. 1965. *Collected Works of Paul Valéry.* Bollingen Series, vol. 45. New York: Pantheon Books.

Pellegrino, E.D. 1979. "Reconstruction of Medical Morality." *Journal of Medicine and Philosophy* 4: 32-56.

Part II:
Physicians and Patients

The Attending Physician
as a Central Figure

Otto E. Guttentag

I am proud and grateful that this conference is being held in my honor. My merit, as far as I can see it, is my mulishness or stubbornness—my doggedness in proclaiming to academic medicine the significance of the care of individual patients. I am compelled to defend the importance of individual health against those diagnostic taxonomists and basic scientists who, in the enthusiasm for their own work, may sometimes venture beyond the limits of their disciplines.

No exchange of thoughts on a topic concerning the medical profession could be closer to my professional heart than that of this conference: the axioms of practicing physicians, the cognitive premises under which they do or should work, and the practical obligations they have to fulfill. Such an evaluation is indeed a demand of our turbulent times, which are as turbulent, I believe, as those of the second through fourth centuries A.D. It is also fortunate that this conference is interdisciplinary, for like any other discipline, medicine needs to analyze its philosophical premises in order not to fall prey to dogmatic and unreflective empiricism.

ORIENTATION

In addressing my assigned topic, "The Attending Physician as a Central Figure," I will not provide any new analyses, but will expand on matters I have discussed in the past (1949, 1950, 1959, 1960, 1966, 1969, 1978). Let me begin by identifying my position and methodological orientation.

First, I speak from an ideal or purely conceptual perspective, that is, from the standpoint of the attending physician as I visualize him, rather than from an experiential standpoint which treats the physician as a statistical average. My specific occupational perspective is that of a reflective medical educator who has been an attending physician and who continues to identify completely with the attending physician's attitude, that is, with the attitude of a person who responds positively to a fellow human being's cry, consciously or implicitly addressed to him, "Help me in the care of my health." In Dr. Pellegrino's terms, I concentrate on "philosophy *in* medicine," not philosophy "*of* medicine" (Pellegrino 1976). My focus is on the meaning of the term *intervention* from the standpoint of the attending physician.

When I say that I identify completely with the perspective of the attending physician, I stress that I examine the axioms of the physician not from the standpoint of a reflective onlooker, but from that of a reflective member of the community of attending physicians. This means that I do not speak from the perspective of a consulting physician, clinical investigator, sociologist, or bioethicist. Detached and objectifying onlookers are an effective and welcome antidote to the intrusion of self-serving egotism, but participants are the best persons to delineate the intricacy of the task (Tillich 1952).

In terms of methodology, my orientation is both pragmatic and phenomenological-existential. It is pragmatic because I do not try to interpret why certain things (which I may deplore and want to change) are as they are, nor do I try to delineate their historical genesis. Instead, I focus on the same area and problems covered by the current sources of pragmatic information, the three standard textbooks of internal medicine: *Cecil's Textbook of Medicine* (1979), *Harrison's Principles of Internal Medicine* (1980), and *The Principles and Practice of Medicine* (Harvey 1976). In their introductory chapters, these three volumes focus on the clinical approach to the patient in the broadest sense.

My approach is phenomenological-existential, for I take very seriously Husserl's famous dictum, to "return to the things themselves" (Husserl 1965). More concretely, I will elucidate certain clinical concepts and orientations that are usually either taken for granted or discussed in a remote manner—concepts and orientations such as those of health and disease and the single disease or clinical entity. These will be related to a concept of the nature of man and to man's relationship to human and nonhuman beings. Both the clinical concepts and the clinical orientation will be viewed in the framework of the ultimate irreducible categories of our experience, such as "I-ness" and "it-ness," freedom and determinism, consciousness and vitality.

Such an approach, which starts from scratch, offers rich benefits: it serves as a powerful prophylactic against lazy routine and blind dogma, and it provides a common denominator, a common meeting ground and point of departure, for all attitudes and paths in the field of medicine. After analyzing some of the axioms of the attending physician, I shall make some small and very simple, yet I think significant, pedagogical recommendations that are not merely uncomfortable appendages to the medical curriculum.

Before turning to my view of the attending physician as a central figure, a few explanatory remarks are in order. First, if my topic had been designed to comply with the parlance of the medical anthropologists, it might have been entitled "The Western Healer as a Central Figure." However, because recent developments in nonestablishment Western medicine have expanded the definition of *healer* to include nonphysicians, I prefer the customary term, *attending physician*.

Second, rather than saying "my attitude is that of an attending physician," it would be more precise to say "I have decided to adopt this attitude." I believe that contemporary Western medicine involves a type of healing that potentially and actually exceeds all other approaches in maintaining that optimal status of selfhood we call "being healthy" and in eliminating that reduced status of selfhood we call "being sick." The ever-spreading acceptance of Western healership supports this view. The medical anthropologist Dunn (1976) recommended that this approach be called "cosmopolitan" healership. The creation of the physician, the division of the duties of the shaman into ministry and physicianship, and, with this division, the localization of the status of being healthy or sick into the realm of nonmoral or "natural" dynamics is, of course, the essence of this healership.

Finally, it is appropriate to say something about the assumption that the viewpoint of the attending physician is central. No one can reasonably doubt that medicine is primarily and ultimately a "utilitarian" discipline, as the editors of the Harrison textbook (1980) express it. Physicians who are not ethically accountable for the care of patients do not confront medicine in this way. Thus, the *attending* physician is doubtless the central figure. But it is reasonable to ask whether the attending physician is expected to serve as a personal physician to a single fellow human being or to a community as a whole, for example, as a public health officer. Obviously, the obligations and tasks of the attending physician differ in these two situations, even though they have in common a concern for the health care of human beings. As McDermott correctly notes in *Cecil's Textbook of Medicine* (1979), both types of attending physicians are necessary. However, from the standpoint of human existence (the perspective from which I speak) it is the individual patient, and not the group, who is the primary and ultimate point of reference. Thus, it is the personal physician who represents the more basic form of the two types of attending physicians. I shall concentrate, therefore, on the axioms of the personal physician.

WHAT IS MEDICINE?

Let me describe how these issues are addressed in a seminar, "Axiomatics of Western Healership (physicianship)," which is offered to medical students and graduate students as an elective.[1] The seminar begins by raising the question: "What is medicine all about in terms of our immediate perception (*Anschauung*)?" A definition of medicine is evolved that is broad enough so that nonphysicians and physicians alike can agree on it, yet precise enough to bring the physician-patient encounter into central focus. The definition is that medicine deals with the care of the health of human beings by human beings. The seminar continues by examining and developing the characteristics of each element in the definition. What do we mean by *care*? By *care of health*? What is meant by *health*, and, particularly, *health of human beings*? Who are we human beings, the ultimate units and concern of medicine? What does the phrase *of human beings, by human beings* imply for the physician-patient relationship? The elements of the definition provide a solid frame of reference for delineating the tasks, recognizing the obligations, and organizing the thoughts of the attending physician.

When I raise the question "What is medicine all about in terms of our immediate perception?", the first answer to emerge is usually "care of health of human beings." One then raises the question "Who takes care, care by whom?" The answer emerges: "By human beings," that is, you and me. I find it amazing—and probably, I fear, an incrimination of present medical education—that every time "by human beings" is added, the students appear as if awakened from slumber. They become excitedly aware of both a fact and an ensuing question; they immediately realize that both are of fundamental significance for their chosen field, and they are apparently confronted with them for the first time in their education. The fact is that patients and physicians are fellow beings, and we physicians can know no more or less about the subjects of our concern than we know about ourselves. To put it another way, the physician-patient relationship is ontologically different from that of a maintenance engineer to a machine or a veterinarian to an animal. The question is, "Who are we human beings?"

While it may seem absurd to try to answer this question in one or two seminar hours, without a characterization of the ultimate units who are asking for and providing medical care, any discussion of medical care is incomplete. However, if we remember that Western healership localizes the states of health and sickness in the "natural" realm, the notion of absurdity fades. To answer the question, a modification of Tillich's (1962) characterization is used: Man is a structured, multiform, multiphasic physical being of "finite freedom," interrelated with a world. Clumsy as the phrase may be in its experiential immediacy, it is broad enough to satisfy any interpreter of the nature of man who is of good will, yet at the same time succinct enough to pinpoint man's nature in a way that illuminates the effort of healership.

The words *physical, multiform,* and *multiphasic* need no detailed elaboration. They refer, respectively, to the experience of ourselves as beings of mass and extension, of storage and transmission of energy (in other words as machinelike beings) to the experience of our dissimilarities, and to our experience of the sequential developmental character of our nature, that is, the various stages of our being, implying an ultimate fulfillment. "Man is a Zeitgestalt" (von Uexküll 1928). The phrase "interrelated with a world" refers to man's intrinsic involvement with his natural and social environment.

The word *freedom* in this context refers to a human as a conscious, reflective, responsible being, a being of conscience, aware of moral issues. Freedom is the essence of what we call personhood, the most articulate form of subjectivity. *Subjectivity* means the phenomena of selfhood, inwardness, autonomy, and spontaneity that characterize the differences between biological and nonbiological physical structures. Biological beings are those physical objects of our experience that can be adequately described only by the term *subjects* rather than *objects*.

The word *finite* refers to our experience of the limitation of our being, of our knowledge both theoretical and practical, and especially of what we call death,[2] the total, inevitable, and unpredictable loss of self, with the implications these phenomena have for our spiritual and moral self-fulfillment (Tillich 1962). The word *of* in the phrase *physical beings of finite freedom*, refers to the polar, not composite, dualism of our nature; in other words, a dualism, like the polar structure of the earth or a magnet, in which the whole precedes the two antithetic propensities.

This characterization of the nature of human beings is used as the background for assessing the other fundamental concepts used in the definition of medicine. Health and disease stand for the maximal and reduced (as distinct from restricted) fulfillment of the most basic and inescapable (prereflective and premoral) conditions of a physical being of finite autonomy. Referring to different states of individual human existence, the terms *health* and *disease* are of theological and sociological significance. They indicate the maximal and reduced capacity of man's inescapable creaturely condition to adjust to norms constructed by dogma or law. *Care* refers to concerned and informed intervention for the good of the other; *care of health*, obviously, to such intervention in regard to health.

THE PHYSICIAN-PATIENT ENCOUNTER

Brief as it is, this characterization of medicine provides an adequate frame of reference for an analysis of the nature and structure of the physician-patient encounter. In an earlier paper, "Care of the Healthy and Sick from the Attending Physician's Perspective" (1978), I discuss the nature of that encounter in detail. One essential feature of the physician-patient relationship is that it is fiducial and ultimately person oriented. It is not contractual-legal in a businesslike sense of promising a result, nor is it fiducial and construct-thing oriented.

In interpersonal relationships, man's freedom manifests itself as the impossibility of being grasped, captured. The other is always ultimately elusive: *Individuum est ineffabile*, a being of unfathomable privacy and inwardness; thus the fiducial character of the relationship. By emphasizing that the relationship is oriented toward persons and not toward things, I wish to underscore the difference between the fields of concern of physician and lawyer. Physicians and lawyers may be considered equals in terms of existential effort, of dyadic solidarity with those who call for help. But statutory law—crimes—can be classified quite rigidly, and punishment is exactly and closely tied to crimes. However, what physicians call a single disease—a concept to which I shall shortly return—is something very fluid and ideal. Despite all the knowledge at his command and the carefulness of his proceedings, a physician may see a minor wound become the portal of death. Textbook descriptions of diseases are not basically social constructs; they are manifestations of our finitude. Indeed, the more physicians advance in insight (the more they "know"), the less they are inclined to translate diagnoses into disease labels.

Turning to the structure of the physician-patient encounter, please recall first that the expressions *being healthy* and *being sick* refer to modes of biological existence, that is, to man's basic inescapable (prereflective and premoral) condition; the second, that man's nature is indivisible and differentiated, but not composite. Thus, the physician concerned with the care of the healthy and sick does not focus on man's intellectual and moral nature. If I am on call, I must take care of my wife's murderer who was wounded when apprehended. Physicians are concerned with the intellectual and moral formulations of their patients only when they affect good health; for example, when fanaticism exacerbates high blood pressure, or, conversely, when changes in intellectual and moral functioning (sluggish intellectual activity) are caused by a disease (such as hypothyroidism), or when a difference in personality structure presents an insurmountable challenge to physician-patient fellowship. But this focus on man's prerational and premoral conditions does not entitle the physician to ignore the "higher" anthropological aspects of medical care. The only adequate medical model is the anthropological-medical model, viewing man as a being of finite freedom, not merely of finite autonomy.[3]

Von Gebsattel (1953, 1954) articulated the structure of the physician-patient encounter by dividing it into three stages. Augmenting and slightly modifying his characterization, they may be called

1. The stage of responsive fellowship: the primary subjective stage of receptive participation. Listening; history-taking in the patient's words but in the professional framework. Ethics of receptive participation.

2. The stage of estrangement (detachment): the objective stage. Nosography and the concept of *a* disease, the clinical entity. Ethics of expertise.

3. The stage of personal communication: the final subjective stage of reciprocal participation. The ethical element in the physician-patient relationship.

The first and third stages deal essentially with the ethics of interhuman communication in medical care. Regarding the first stage, I will mention only the intricacy of taking the patient's history. By this I mean not only the difficulty of taking a history *in* the patient's words and *from* the patient's point of view and transforming this knowledge into the professional frame of reference, but also the need for the physician to be alert to and able to interpret the patient's linguistics, phonetics, and body language. We are much indebted to Cassell and Skopek (1977) for the exploration of this field, and to Laín Entralgo (1956) for his emphasis on patience, as well as his reminder that the German clinician von Leyden (1832-1910) used to tell his students: "The first act of the physician's caring consists of shaking the hand of the patient."

The third stage deals with the relationship of patient and physician as persons in all the complexity of individual metaphysics and the dialectical tensions of partnership. Consider, for example, the obligation of telling the truth. The patient as a fellow human being has every right to know the truth about his or her biological condition. Yet other considerations enter into the fulfillment of this obligation: the mutual influences of the somatic and the personal poles (the dualism) of our nature, and our anxiety concerning death—actual death. No one can be objective toward his or her own body (Jaspers 1963). Telling an unwelcome truth to the unprepared is as ill-conceived as trying to hide the truth from the prepared. In the words of the great clinician Thomas Addis (1948), "Honesty with patients requires thought and discipline and effort."

The Clinical Entity

I need to deal at some length with the second stage, the stage of estrangement or "objectivation," with its emphasis on the physical-biological dimension of man's nature. This is not, however, because of its ethical demands, nor because of the attitude taken by some nonphysicians who view this stage in isolation and characterize it, with the phrase "medical model," as an interhuman relationship restricted to this phase. Such use of the phrase is ill-conceived. As Laín Entralgo has pointed out, this phase is very rarely isolated in actual medical care. Instead, I must examine the second stage in some detail because of its fundamental general concept, the concept of the single or specific disease, the "clinical entity." Faber, the great Danish clinician, called this the concept without which attending physicians "cannot live, cannot speak, cannot act" (1930). But this concept has received very little systematic attention in the recent past. Although the epitomes of clinical thought, the textbooks of medicine, are outstanding in describing what are characterized as single diseases (e.g., peptic ulcer, glomerular nephritis, typhoid fever), they never delineate the basic common denominator of those entities. Can one imagine a textbook of histology without a chapter on the cell or a textbook of physics or chemistry without a chapter on the atom?

The absence of attention in medicine to the concept of the "clinical entity" is unfortunate, because it deprives nonphysicians of any insight into the attending physician's organization of thought, and it entices medical students and young physicians to think in terms of labels instead of more basic categories. Furthermore, and of no less importance, every older physician knows that what is considered today to be one disease may tomorrow be considered several, and vice versa. Similarly, in terms of broader medical history—and the following is most important—what is considered to be the nature and structure of the concept of the single disease or clinical entity at any given period may yield to another perception of this conception at another. Thus, lack of awareness of the basic concept of clinical thought stifles not only genuine reflective observation within a given frame of reference, but also genuine reflective observation concerning the frame of reference itself. For all these reasons, a brief delineation of the concept of the clinical entity, as we view it today, is important.

First, it should be noted that the concept of the single disease or clinical entity is a typological concept, a concept of higher order that tries to unify the view of several independent solitary units, several sick patients. However, although the most individual aspect of man's nature recedes in the description of the clinical entity, it never disappears. It represents a person in all his or her complexity as faced by the physician.

In the immediate confrontation with the patient, the concept focuses on what concerns the patient most: first, the predicted course of the reduced state of the patient's psychosomatic freedom of action, and second, the physician's ability to intervene. The concept of the single disease or clinical entity tries to answer these questions as precisely as a typological concept can. In turn, the concept of the clinical entity is the attending physician's most basic tool for providing a concrete answer to the patient's cry for help concerning his health. For physicians, the concept of the single disease provides an aggregation of some phenomena of a sick organism, some events of the organism's environment, and a history of these occurrences that can be viewed as a unit, a specific anthropologic-biological pattern. To paraphrase Rather (1961), this is a unit based broadly on some more or less certain and orderly recurring features of man's most basic being-in-the-world, formulated as precisely as possible in terms of an interpretation of the nature and structure of this dimension. Today the clinical entity or single disease concept is formulated or patterned by visualizing the phenomena and their "Zeitgestalt" in their interdependence: formal and mechanical as well as rationally causal and, in the psychiatric field especially, understandable interdependence.[4]

Therapy and Research

Returning to the physician-patient encounter, I wish to touch briefly on the issues of therapy in relation to the justification of therapeutic recommendations, and research done by the attending physician versus that done by the medical or clinical scientist.

Concerning therapy, the 2500-year-old adage, "First, do no harm," is still the admonition that overrides all else. Subservient to this principle, and in relation to the nature of man and the view of medicine as a utilitarian discipline, four approaches to therapy may be differentiated. They are (*a*) the antipathic approach, directed toward eliminating some recognized malfunction (most forms of pharmacological and surgical intervention exemplify this approach); (*b*) the biological approach, aimed at reinforcing the human organism's self-sustaining capabilities, for example, methods of relaxation training and immunotherapy; (*c*) the personal approach, aimed at eliciting existential acceptance by the patient of less rigid and incongruous limits of human freedom than a patient perceives (psychotherapy through "the word"); and (*d*) the utilitarian approach, usually called the "simply empirical."

Which do we use? To make the choice the physician looks for that therapy for which positive results have been confirmed by controlled experiments, that is, confirmed by experiments presenting the greatest challenge to the causal nexus between the specific interventional procedure and the hoped-for result. Although difficulties of choice may arise under any circumstances—*individuum est ineffabile*—they reach their climax when the therapeutic methods fail and the patient asks for one or more of the generally unapproved therapeutic approaches. Although he may disassociate himself from any particular approach, the attending physician would be careless and dogmatic to stand in the way of the patient, provided there is reason to believe that the approach requested does not harm and that its performers are honest in presenting their claims. The physician would be equally careless, ignoring his Western background of reason and logic, if he allowed those approaches to be taught to his students when their advocates were unwilling to submit their claims to the demands of critical evaluation. In other words, it is the failure to submit to the demands of testing, rather than the underlying concepts themselves, that leads many unestablished therapeutic approaches to be labeled as cults.

Finally, I want to touch on the problem of research in clinical medicine, that is, research in the care of health from the standpoint of the attending physician. Although individual physicians have differing degrees of interest in research, medical students must be taught to view the problems of medical obligation not only in terms of current knowledge but also in terms of the search for better solutions than those offered today. The full experience of medical concern requires the imparting of current knowledge and, at the same time, the dissatisfaction that this knowledge is so limited.

CONCLUSION

This paper has explored the central themes of my seminar, "Axiomatics of Western Healership." The starting point is a characterization of medicine as the "care of health of human beings by human beings." This is followed by the attempt to delineate the individual elements of this characterization: human beings, health and disease, care, and the nature and structure of the physician-patient relationship in terms of Western post-Christian culture. These studies provide a basis for understanding the frame of reference of the attending physician and for developing his axioms. They provide a framework for the evaluation of a medical attitude in general, as well as for an individual physician's appraisal of himself. Medical students gain a clearer recognition of the relationships among the various subjects of the medical curriculum, as well as an understanding of the organization of medical training as a whole. The seminar aids medical students to understand their general cultural environment through the analysis of the concept of the physician as it has emerged in Western culture.

My first recommendation is that a course such as the one outlined here be given to all first-year medical students or, even earlier, to undergraduate students interested in going to medical school. (I made this recommendation in the *Journal of Medical Education* in 1960.)

Second, I would also propose that attempts to foster the personalistic aspects of medical care in medical education be more precisely focused than they are at present on the pragmatic, utilitarian aspects of medical care. Such an emphasis, with a course on the axioms of Western establishment healership as background, does not deprive of its intrinsic value any topic on which such attempts may focus. By a greater emphasis on pragmatic, utilitarian aspects I mean, for example, that courses in medical anthropology, dealing with non-Western systems of healership or nonestablishment approaches to medical care, should also allow Western attending physicians to assess the assets and liabilities of the medical approaches discussed. Courses in the history of therapy and preventive medicine—the primary and ultimate core topics of the entire medical effort—should also be offered; if not taught by physicians, they should certainly include discussion by physicians of the approaches presented. The same holds true for courses in ethics or literature. Why should a medical student, already burdened with a heavy schedule, be interested in literature courses not specifically geared to the medical curriculum? The answer is that such courses could readily be addressed to subjects of medical interest, for example, the role of the attending physician's silent partner, death? Readings of Plato's "The Death of Socrates," Tolstoi's *The Death of Ivan Il'ich*, Chekhov's "The Bet," or Rilke's poem in the *Book of Hours* which begins, "Oh, Lord, grant each his own, his death indeed, the dying which out of that life evolved in which he once had meaning, love and need ... ," would certainly attract medical students and not be "uncomfortable appendages to the medical curriculum."

In summary, then, a seminar aimed at elucidating the axioms of Western healership (physicianship) in their timelessness and concreteness offers several significant advantages:

1. It deals with the core of the discipline, not with adornments; it is utterly pragmatic.
2. It alerts the physicians of a given period not to become infatuated with themselves or fall prey to routine and dogma.
3. It introduces medical students to the spirit of their discipline.
4. It familiarizes nonmedical people with the intricacy and weight

of the attending physician's response: "Yes, I will help you in the care of your health."

In short, such a course or seminar would enable prospective doctors and patients to understand the attending physician's motto: *Salus aegroti suprema lex*—the welfare of the patient is the supreme law.

Notes

1. For topics outside my field of competence, I am grateful for the assistance of Prof. Edward W. Hobbs and others from the Graduate Theological Union, Berkeley, California.

"Axiomatics of Western Healership" is a seminar offered at the University of California, San Francisco.

2. Death as fulfillment is a regulative principle and must, of course, be differentiated from actual death, which removes the possibilities of further development that always appear to be present (Guttentag 1959, 1969).

3. Physicians considered to be great by every member of the profession have never, throughout history, abandoned this attitude (if I understand Professor Laín Entralgo [1956, 1969] correctly), except perhaps in the case of sociological attitudes concerning social classes or ethnic groups.

4. This interdependence is seen in four areas: environment (see Table 1 on page 120); biological diversity (see Table 2 on page 121); topography, both structural and functional (see Table 3 on page 121); and pathology (see Table 4 on page 122). We know very little of the biological diversity factor. It refers to the patient's "constitution," that is, the "undestructable typological attempt" to grasp "the infinite whole of somato-psychic life in its un-understandable foundations" (Jaspers 1963). Published material familiar to physicians includes Behnke et al. (1953); Gertler and White (1954); Guttentag (1966); Kretschmer (1936, 1977); and Sheldon (1940, 1942, 1949, 1954). With regard to the topographic functional factor, it is important not to confuse functional thinking with clinical thinking. Clinical thinking is prognostic thinking; functional thinking is *part of* clinical thinking and does not, in itself, imply prognosis. The interrelationships of these factors are represented in Figure 1 on page 123.

Table 1. Environmental Factors

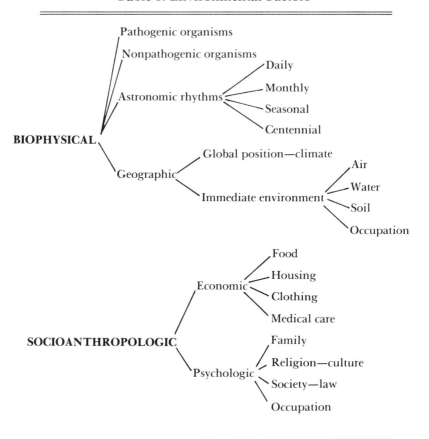

a. Modified from unpublished material of S.P. Lucia.

Table 2. Biological Diversity Factor

Anthropological Component	Freedom: man's conscious autonomy
Developmental-Constitutional Component	Age
	Constitutional patterns
	Differentiation by structural characteristics
	Differentiation by functional characteristics (including reactions to drugs)

Table 3. Topographical Factor (Structural and Functional)[a]

Integumentary	Renal
Musculoskeletal	Genital
Bronchopulmonary	Ductless Glands
Cardiovascular	Cerebral—Nervous
Blood and General Body Fluids	Chromosomes—Genes
Gastroenteric	Combination of Systems
	Psychological—Personal

Reserve capacity: the amount of specific work an organ is capable of carrying out—over and above what it is actually doing—without incurring any irreversible functional or structural change.

a. Modified from *Standard Nomenclature of Disease* (1942), and from textbooks of medicine by Cecil (1979), Harrison (1980), and Harvey et al. (1976).

Table 4. Pathological Factor (Somatic Aberrations)[a,b]

Structural aberrations

Chromosomes and genes	Disturbances in chromosome numbers, organization, structure	Abnormal number Translocation Deletion or duplication of chromosomal parts
	Disturbances in gene (codon) structure: intragenic or intergenic	Deletion, addition or substitution of nucleotides
Cells	Regressive processes	Atrophy Rearrangement (swelling, degeneration) Substitution Necrosis
	Progressive processes	Hypertrophy Regeneration Metaplasia
Tissue Organization	Inflammation	Degeneration Exudative Productive Specific
	Regeneration	Healing by primary intention Healing by secondary intention (granulation)
	Atypical hyperplasias (tumors)	
Organic union	Disturbances in circulation Endocrine disturbances Fevers Death	

Functional aberrations

Relative or absolute malfunction	Hypofunction Hyperfunction Dysfunction Disturbance of regulation	

---

a. Psychological personal aberrations are also part of the pathological factor. One descriptive list is found on pp. 61-65 of May, Angel, and Ellenberger (1959).

b. Modified from Oertel (1927) and from unpublished data of P.F. Kelly.

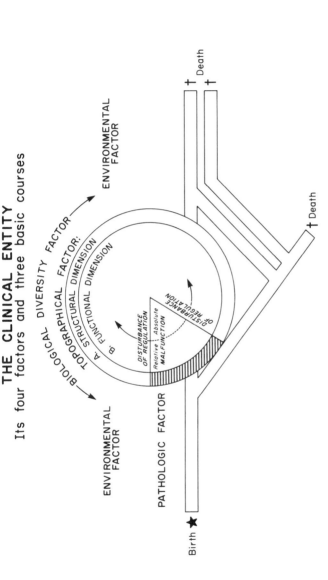

Figure 1. The circle and its contents represent a living organism from birth (star) to death (cross on right side). The oblique line downward ending with a cross represents a course leading to premature death, the line joining the horizontal line represents the course of a completely regressive disease, the line going toward the horizontal line, then turning parallel to the horizontal line represents the course of a partly regressive stationary disease. The area around the circle represents the environmental factor. The biologic diversity factor is meant to be represented by the size of the circle. Although this circle runs from birth to death, there is a play within the play, namely that of pathology, denoted by the pathological factor and the area of the functional dimension belonging to the pathological factor.

Bibliography

Addis, T. 1948. *Glomerular Nephritis: Diagnosis and Treatment.* New York: Macmillan.

Behnke, A.R., Osserman, E.F., and Welham, W.C. 1953. "Lean Body Mass." *Archives of Internal Medicine* 91: 585-601.

Boss, M. 1979. *Existential Foundations of Medicine and Psychology,* translated by S. Conway and A. Cleaves. New York: Aronson.

Cassell, E.J., and Skopek, L. 1977. "Language as a Tool in Medicine: Methodology and Theoretical Framework." *Journal of Medical Education* 52: 197-203.

Cecil's Textbook of Medicine. 1979. 15th ed. Edited by P.B. Beeson, W. McDermott, and J.B. Wyngaarden. Philadelphia: W.B. Saunders.

Childress, J.F. 1985. "Rights and Responsibilities of Patients: A Commentary on Pedro Laín Entralgo," pp. 145-150 in this volume.

Dunn, F.L. 1976. "Traditional Asian Medicine and Cosmopolitan Medicine as Adaptive Systems." In *Asian Medical Systems: A Comparative Study,* edited by C. Leslie. Berkeley: University of California Press.

Engelhardt, H.T., Jr. 1985. "Causal Accounts in Medicine: A Critique," pp. 73-81 in this volume.

Faber, K. 1930. *Nosography: The Evolution of Clinical Medicine in Modern Times.* New York: Hoeber.

Gertler, D.M., and White, P.D. 1954. *Coronary Heart Disease in Young Adults.* Cambridge, MA: Harvard University Press.

Guttentag, O.E. 1949. "On the Clinical Entity." *Annals of Internal Medicine* 31: 484-96.

_____ . 1950. "Two Diagrams on the Clinical Entity." *Journal of Pediatrics* 37: 530-34.

_____ . 1959. "The Meaning of Death in Clinical Theory." *Stanford Medical Bulletin* 17: 165-70.

_____ . 1960. "A Course Entitled 'The Medical Attitude': An Orientation in the Foundations of Medical Thought." *Journal of Medical Education* 35: 903-07.

_____. 1966. "Homeopathy in the Light of Modern Pharmacology." *Clinical Pharmacology and Therapeutics* 7: 425-28.

_____. 1969. "Medical Humanism: A Redundant Phrase." *Pharos* 32: 12-15.

_____. 1978. "Care of the Healthy and the Sick from the Attending Physician's Perspective: Envisioned and Actual." In *Organism, Medicine and Metaphysics*, edited by S.F. Spicker. Dordrecht, The Netherlands: D. Reidel Publishing Co.

Harrison's Principles of Internal Medicine. 1980. 9th ed. Edited by K.J. Isselbacher, R.D. Adams, E. Braunwald, R.G. Petersdorf, and J.D. Wilson. New York: McGraw-Hill.

Harvey, A.M., Johns, R.J., Owens, A.H., Jr., and Ross, R.J. 1976. *The Principles and Practice of Medicine*. 19th ed. New York: Appleton-Century-Crofts.

Husserl, E. 1965. "Philosophy as a Rigorous Science." In *Edmund Husserl: Phenomenology and the Crisis of Philosophy*, translated by Q. Lauer. New York: Harper and Row.

Jaspers, K. 1963. *General Psychopathology*. 7th ed. Translated by J. Hoenig and M.W. Hamilton. Manchester, England: Manchester University Press.

Kretschmer, E. 1936. *Physique and Character: An Investigation of the Nature of Constitution and of the Theory of Temperament*. 2d ed. New York: Harcourt, Brace.

_____. 1977. *Körperbau und Charakter: Untersuchungen zum Konstitutionsproblem und zur lehre von der Temperamenten*. Berlin: Springer-Verlag.

Laín Entralgo, P. 1956. "Mind and Body." In *Psychosomatic Pathology: A Short History of the Evolution of Medical Thought*. Translated by A.M. Espinosa, Jr. New York: Kenedy and Sons.

_____. 1969. *Doctor and Patient*. Translated by F. Partidge. New York: McGraw-Hill.

_____. 1985. "What Does the Word *Good* Mean in *Good Patient?*", pp. 127-143 in this volume.

May, R., Angel, E., and Ellenberger, N.F. 1959. *Existence*. New York: Basic Books.

Oertel, H. 1927. *Outlines of Pathology*. Montreal: Renouf Publishing Co.

Pellegrino, E.D. 1976. "Philosophy of Medicine: Problematic and Potential." *Journal of Medicine and Philosophy* 1: 5-31.

Rather, L.J. 1961. "The Disease Entity." *Stanford Medical Bulletin* 19: 142-45.

Reiser, S.J. 1985. "Environmental versus Biological Causation in Medicine: A Commentary on Max Black," pp. 197-201 in this volume.

Schaffner, K.F. 1985. "Modeling Clinical Medicine: A Commentary on Mark Siegler," pp. 43-58 in this volume.

Sheldon, W.H. 1940. *The Varieties of Human Physique: An Introduction to Constitutional Psychology*. New York: Harper and Brothers.

_____ . 1942. *The Varieties of Temperament: A Psychology of Constitutional Differences*. New York: Harper and Brothers.

_____ . 1949. *Varieties of Delinquent Youth: An Introduction to Constitutional Psychiatry*. New York: Harper and Brothers.

_____ . 1954. *Atlas of Men: A Guide for Somatotyping the Adult Male of All Ages*. New York: Harper and Brothers.

Standard Nomenclature of Disease. 1942. Chicago: American Medical Association.

Tillich, P. 1952. *The Courage to Be*. New Haven: Yale University Press.

_____ . 1962. "What Is Basic in Human Nature." *American Journal of Psychoanalysis* 22: 115-21.

Toulmin, S. 1953. *The Philosophy of Science: An Introduction*. New York: Harper and Brothers.

_____ . 1985. "Causation and the Locus of Medical Intervention," pp. 59-72 in this volume.

von Gebsattel, V.E. 1953. "Zur Sinnstruktur der aerztlichen Haltung." *Studium Generale* 6: 461-71.

_____ . 1954. *Prolegomena einer medizinischen Anthropologie*. Berlin: Springer-Verlag.

von Uexküll, J. 1928. *Theoretische Biologie zweite gänzlich neu bearbeitete Auflage*. Berlin: Verlag von Julius Springer.

What Does the Word *Good* Mean in *Good Patient?*

Pedro Laín Entralgo

In analyzing what it means to be a good patient, two initial questions arise. What does the adjective *good* mean before a generic noun? Is its meaning the same in expressions such as *good watch, good horse, good poet, good patient?* Let us consider these questions briefly.

Before any generic noun, the adjective *good* denotes the condition of a thing that fully and completely fulfills its own being. A good watch fully and completely fulfills the essential being of the object that we call *watch;* the same thing would have to be said mutatis mutandis of the expressions *good horse, good poet,* and *good patient,* at least by a preliminary analysis. However, is the "full and complete realization of being" itself the same in every case I have just cited? Surely not.

A good watch is one that indicates, in a precise and clear way, the course of cosmic time: this and nothing else. Everything else about it—the value of the material from which it is made, the artistic excellence of its workmanship—is a purely accessory judgment. The raison d'être of the watch, a human artifact, has a character both clear-cut and univocal; as a result, our minds can grasp the full understanding of it.

Can we say the same thing about the expression *good horse?* Not at all, since the horse—a natural entity diversely utilized by man and not constructed by him—can be good in two senses. First of all, a good horse is a horse in which the properties and features of the species *Equus caballus* are fully and completely fulfilled. This does not mean that a horse that does not fulfill these conditions perfectly cannot be called good by someone who obtains from it some special service, such as aggressiveness in combat or endurance on long marches. Thus, a horse can be good zoologically (good as itself) and good socially (good in its occasional service to man); a medieval scholar would say good *simpliciter* and good *secundum quid*.

The case of the good poet is more complex. Following the preceding formula, the good poet would be one who fully and completely fulfills his own being as a poet. But since a poet is a poet only insofar as he or she creates poetry, and since this poetry can itself be judged by its quality, *good poet* may mean—if one prefers another formula— the person who writes good poetry. This raises several questions that are not easy to resolve, such as (1) What constitutes good poetry? Are there, perhaps, objective and universal criteria that apply? Undoubtedly not. Personal or group preferences and criteria will result in the application of the word *good* to dissimilar poems. (2) A poem is the result of the personal creative act of its author; it is not a biological response to an external stimulus. Might not an examination of the creative act of the poet—the very manner by which poems are created— uncover particular ways of being a good or a bad poet? The poet fully becomes one when, after having written a poem, it is accepted and incorporated as part of one's personal existence; that is to say, the poet does not try to burn it or to forget it. This establishes a new point of view for formulating or shaping the judgment of what it means to be a good poet.

Let us come, finally, to the subject at hand, that of the patient whom we may or may not call a "good patient" or a "good sick person." Applying the proposed formula, we may begin by saying that the good patient is the person who, as a patient, fully and completely fulfills his essential being. But just what constitutes being a patient or being sick? Only by answering this question can we understand what it is for someone to fully and completely fulfill their essential being as a patient. Two complementary answers are possible, depending upon whether we see "being a patient" (or "being sick") as an anomalous state in the life of the person suffering illness or as a correctable deficiency. Let us examine the answers in order.

ILLNESS AS AN ANOMALOUS STATE

The mode of life we call "sickness" can be understood from the point of view of an observer (i.e., as the mode of life of the sick person who stands before me) or from the point of view of the patient (i.e., as the peculiarity of my life when I am ill). This second point of view is the one which principally concerns us.

Basic Aspects of Sickness

"I am sick," or "I feel sick." When a person speaks this way, what does he mean? Just this: that somehow, in living his life, he has encountered a strange, anomalous moment that the society to which he belongs customarily calls "being sick." The particular modes of this feeling can be very diverse: for example, feeling pain in some part of one's body, having fever, dizziness, being paralyzed, vomiting, having swellings or hallucinations, seeing a change in the color of one's skin. All these are only the concrete manifestations of a generic feeling to which the following seven elementary experiences belong: invalidism, discomfort, threat, being tied to one's body, solitude, anomaly, and the opportunity to act.

Invalidism. Invalidism is the total or partial incapacity to carry out some of the functions of human life, such as moving about in space, seeing, thinking, speaking, and eating. Being sick is, then, a state of "not-being-able-to" or a "being-able-to-with-difficulty." From this results some of the names by which illness is known in various languages: for example, *infirmitas, asthénia, disease.* Understood in this generic sense, it hardly seems necessary to point out that invalidism does not always mean paralysis or absence of function: for example, vomiting prevents eating, hand tremors prevent one from writing, and an obsessive mental compulsion interrupts thinking. The experience of invalidism may put whoever experiences it in a state of necessity, a state of having to do something with regard to himself.

Discomfort. Discomfort refers to the unpleasant feelings that in different degrees (from slight indisposition to unbearable pain), and in varied forms (from psychic dullness to giddy disorientation), mark the state of illness.

Threat. Threat is the realization that one may be subject to death or to permanent change which brings with it the experience of illness itself, particularly when the threat is intense or persistent.

Being tied to one's body. The sick person may develop the almost unconquerable fixation on his own body. Attention may be drawn to a particular body part that disease has made hypersensitive, to the body as a whole (as in fever), or to nonlocalized psychic symptoms, such as an obsession or a delirious convulsion in which the body's disorder expresses itself.

Solitude. The feeling of isolation that comes with being tied to one's body and to the subjective sensations of the body that are so difficult to communicate (my stomach pain is "mine" and cannot be anyone else's) produces a sense of solitude in the sick person.

Anomaly. Objectively considered, the state of sickness is always "abnormal." Thus, such a state has as its subjective correlative the feeling of anomaly. In comparison to the healthy individuals who surround him, the sick person feels different or abnormal, whether the mode of that difference be inferiority or superiority.

Opportunity to act. Every life state, even the most destructive, presents the person with an opportunity to do something which otherwise could never be done. Thus, it does not matter that sickness never ceases to be a difficult experience or that one may have to endure invalidism, pain, threat, being tied to one's body, solitude, or anomaly; the state of sickness offers the patient the chance to do or even be something new or original. If the state of sickness did not present itself immediately as a call to action, the pathological behavior called "flight into sickness" would not exist.

Let us leave aside the biological mechanisms (e.g., neurophysiological, endocrinological, biochemical, etc.) that result in the "generic feeling of being ill." For our present problem—learning precisely what makes a "good patient"—it is more important to know how the sick person conducts himself in the face of his illness and to determine his attitudes and reactions toward that way of experiencing one's life that we call "being sick."

A person feels that, suddenly or gradually, some part of his being invalids him, pains him, threatens him, obliges him to fix his attention on his body, isolates him, changes him into both a social and biological anomaly. In the face of this disturbance of his life, what will he do? Two distinct reactions can be discerned: one is emotional, the other interpretive.

Emotional Responses

Emotionally, the sick person experiences how this state implants itself in his life and changes the way he lives—according to the social and cultural group to which he belongs, and depending upon what part of his ailment is somatic and psychic *pathos* (i.e., passive suffering of the body and soul). More briefly, he experiences everything to which he, *Homo patiens*, is "being patient."

I cannot present here in any depth the psychology and phenomenology of this suffering, nor can I establish in detail a comprehensive description of the various ways in which it shows itself. Nevertheless, a sketch of the emotional responses to illness might begin with the enumeration of seven basic attitudes.

Fear. The sick person feels fear when seized by the feeling of sickness itself, but above all, in the face of invalidism, pain, threat, and so on. The sick person may experience his fear as depression or as anxiety. Blum (1956) and Feifel (1959) have sensitively discussed the sick person's fear of his illness, while Zborowski (1952) has studied attitudes toward pain.

Rebellion. The sick person rebels more or less intensely and expressively—at times, desperately—against a state that is painfully disturbing, and one which he does not see as being his own fault.

Resigned surrender. Like a willow in a storm, the patient limits himself to giving in to his suffering without protest, enduring it passively.

Active acceptance. The sick person does not rebel against his sickness and is able to accept it as an inevitable vicissitude in the course of his life. However, he does not resign himself to it, and takes action against it by bringing to bear all the resources at hand.

Indifference, apathy. Either as an immediate response (physical lassitude or malaise), or as an expression of deep and vital anguish (Bernbeu 1958; Spitz 1945), or because he believes such conduct to be the best way of being a good patient (Blum 1956; Feifel 1959), the sick person acts in the face of his suffering as if he were indifferent to its possible severe effect on his life.

Neediness. The experience of invalidism that accompanies sickness gives rise to an awareness of living in a "state of necessity." An understanding begins to arise, vague and tenuous in some persons, clear and accusing in others, that the patient must depend on help from others, and, more generally, from a special other.

Childishness. The sick person, as we have just seen, knows himself to be especially in need of help and protection. Even among so-called inner-directed men, this may give rise to attitudes that may properly be called "childish."

Interpretations of Illness

The patient cannot limit himself to feeling his suffering, the psychic weight of his illness; he must also interpret the very fact of his suffering. In one way or another, he must try to make sense of this difficult change of fortune in his life, and also try to understand the place of illness in human life in general. His own psychological makeup, the cultural and social group to which he belongs, and the type of sickness from which he suffers are now, as before, the factors that will orient his interpretations. In my judgment, there are three major kinds of interpretations.

Punishment. In every major culture—Assyria, Babylonia, Israel, Greece (recall the plague in the first Canto of the *Iliad*)—man has believed sickness to be a punishment the sick person must undergo to expiate faults or sins he has committed. This is not some transitory historical interpretation now outmoded by the progressive sophistication of the human intellect. A thorough analysis of the role that guilt plays in the soul of man, consciously or unconsciously, particularly when he is ill, demonstrates that the force of this ancient conception of illness endures in our time.

Chance. From seeing illness as a punishment of the gods, there evolved in ancient Greece an understanding of the morbid accident as a "necessity" of Nature. She, Nature, *physis*, is the "divine," and to her multiform course belongs the possibility of illness (unless the gods intervene). This necessity was conceived along two distinct lines:

first, as "fatal necessity" (*anánkê*), the invincible inevitability of sickness that surges inexorably, against which the actions of men can do nothing; and second, as "chance necessity" (*týkhê*), the sufferings that man's art may dominate, avoid, or cure. "Chance necessity" encompasses the majority of sufferings that the doctor observes.

The growing sophistication of the human mind about its world and the constant progress of the physician's technical skills have relegated to oblivion the concept of falling ill through fatal necessity. However, even in sufferings clearly arising from genetic alterations, modern thought grants general vogue to the idea of chance. This chance is considered to be subject to statistical laws and susceptible to biochemical, biophysical, and psychological explanations. However, such explanations are possible only when the event has already occurred, and can be applied only in retrospect. Calling events "chance" instead of "fatal necessity" does not make their appearance any less enigmatic in the general order of the universe. Except for those who believe in a utopian future where human life would be without sickness, the arising of each episode of illness, its reason for appearing in the cosmos's economy and in the life of whomever suffers it, never ceases to be a painful enigma.

The chance of every episode of illness gives rise to two very distinct, but in no way irreconcilable, attitudes in whoever lives or contemplates it. According to one, the afflictive chance happening that constitutes the morbid accident is lived like a challenge flung in the face of man's inventive and technical powers. A very early example of this is in the Hippocratic writing *De Prisca Medicina*. By the second account, in the pain of illness is seen absurdity, a reality completely incomprehensible and unjustifiable. "Why am I sick? Why do people become sick?" patients ask, never receiving a satisfactory answer. A recent, more extreme example of this attitude is represented by Camus's *The Plague*. Chance, challenge, and absurdity are the three coordinates of the interpretation of sickness peculiar to modern secular man.

Test. Lastly, a person may feel and understand his sickness to be a moral test, in the sense of either merit or distinction. There are some for whom a well-borne sickness is an occasion of merit, in this life or after death. "With regard to the sufferings of the body," wrote Basilius of Caesarea to his friend Hilarion,

> I exhort you to behave with constancy and decency before God, who has called us; because should He see us receive these present things as acts of Grace, He will either calm suffering or affliction, as with Job, or, with great haloes of patience will reward us after this life (Epist. 212,2).

Pascal composed the *Prière pour demander à Dieu le bon usage des maladies*, and Novalis proposed the cultivation of the "art of utilizing illness." And there are others, particularly in secular societies, who see a source of distinction or elegance in the habit of stoically enduring the suffering that sickness brings with it. Recall how a dandy of the Romantic era lived his tuberculosis.

Patients as Agents

The emotional responses to the state of illness—fear, rebellion, resigned surrender, active acceptance, indifference, neediness, childishness—and the simultaneous existential interpretation of illness—as a punishment, an accident of chance, or as a moral test—offer very valuable and important elements for defining what precisely constitutes a good patient. But illness is not simply a sudden and unfortunate vicissitude in the life of the sufferer or a determinant of the kind of suffering (*pathos*) that the sick person must undergo. Rather, the state of sickness (the *nosos*) includes not only passive suffering (*pathos*), as Galenic pathology taught, but is also an active endeavor: *ergon*, the result of a reactive operation, as Sydenham made clear. *Ergon* is not only biological—sickness as a defensive function of the organism (more intense in acute diseases and less in chronic ones)—but is also human and personal *ergon*, although ordinarily in an accessory, subconscious mode. Therefore (and in order not to stray from Greek terminology), the state of sickness is *poiêma*, the production or creation of the subject of the sickness.

The philosopher Zubiri teaches that in the realization of his own being, man is at once agent, actor, and author. He is agent of his muscles' contractions, actor in his life's comedy or drama in society's theater, and author of his comedy's or drama's plot (though never the sole and complete author). But is he only agent, actor, and author? In the most active and creative moments of his life, these three are the notes that appear in the foreground. A moment's thought suffices to show that man is also and simultaneously patient, spectator, and interpreter of himself: patient of his muscular contractions, since he is the one who must feel them; complacent or unhappy spectator of his life's comedy or drama; superficial or profound interpreter, certain or mistaken of the sense that this comedy or drama essentially possesses. When our actions are more imposed from the outside than created from the inside, these last three are the notes that appear in the foreground. Following Freud, pathology discovered that the sick person, in addition to being the patient, spectator, and interpreter of his illness, is also, in some mode and in some measure, agent, author, and actor of that illness.

Certainly the genesis and structure of a neurosis can never be understood without taking into account all aspects of its role in the life of the neurotic; the latter, in effect, is at once patient, spectator, interpreter, agent, actor, and author of the ailment operating within him. Thus, there can be seen a subtle and profound analysis of the symptomatic expression of his illness. This is no less true in illnesses far removed from neurotic modes: cancer, a fracture, arteriosclerosis, infectious disease. How can the sick person's title in them be agent, author, and actor, and not only patient, spectator, interpreter? This occurs through mechanisms more or less immersed in the subconscious psyche, more or less hidden from the mode of being and acting we call "consciousness."

Regarding the genesis of the illness. A fracture is determined primarily by the mechanical forces that have broken the bone. But on occasion and in a subtle way, it is also determined by the hidden operation of personal habits by virtue of which the risk of having accidents capable of producing fractures is very high. Without causal intent, even without awareness, the patient is then coauthor of his ailment. An infectious disease results from chance infection by a microbe—for example, exposure to the yellow fever virus in the course of a tropical expedition—and its consequent pathogenic action in the host. But a detailed examination of the patient's history may reveal that some crisis of life led to an altered capacity to resist this pathogenic organism, and that therefore his person, not merely his biological organism, has participated in the genesis of his sickness. However subordinate and accessory the sick person's participation may be as agent, actor, and author of himself in the genesis of his illness, it is evident that the systematic investigation of such factors has opened an important path toward the understanding of a truly human pathology (Weizseaker 1951).

Regarding the form of the clinical illness. There are many illnesses whose genesis, according to what we know today, is purely biological, or at most biological-social: cancer, for example. But even in these, the role of the patient's person is clear. The sick person's reality, which is not simply biological or organic process, plays a part in the total configuration of the clinical portrait. On one hand, the way that certain symptoms present—for example, hypertension, tachycardia, vomiting, weight loss, and tremors—is qualitatively and quantitatively modified by influences of a personal nature. Any sensible and attentive clinician is capable of noticing that the intensity and presentation of such symptoms are always clearly "personalized," however evident may be the anatomical or biochemical nature of their cause. Let me repeat the formula used before: In addition to being the patient of his symptoms, the sick person is now coauthor of his symptoms. There are also symptoms, on the other hand, determined by subconscious mechanisms, which are symbolic expressions of profound conflicts. This happens particularly in those areas of organic activity in which the final stage is the common terminus of anatomical or patho-physiological changes which are very distinct in themselves. Babin-ski's sign reveals, almost universally, the existence of *one* well-circum-scribed organic change, a lesion of the pyramidal system. In no way can we say the same thing about nausea, tachycardia, constipation, or vertigo. Finally, there are symptoms whose presence in the clinical picture (in a certain way, tacked onto what is essential in it) follow mechanisms of a purely personal order—at times subconscious, at other times semiconscious. Thus, aside from creating suffering (*pathos*), there are one or more paths by which sickness manifests itself (*ergon, poîêma*). Witness typical locution in French medical language: *le malade fait ulcère duodenal* or *une crise d'insuffisance rénal fait*; *fait, makes*, is more profound than one would think at first glance.

Regarding the individualization of the illness. It is in the trinity of *pathos*, *ergon*, and *poîêma* (the kind of suffering that must be undergone, the individual's biological/psychological reaction, the part he has played in the creation of the illness) that illness becomes ultimately and definitively personalized. This is acknowledged whenever the sick person agrees within himself to call it "mine": "my" gastric ulcer, "my" diabetes. In the case of illness, rebellion and resignation are cardinal forms of personalization, though not the only ones. Between St. Francis of Assisi, for whom the affliction caused by an eye disease was "a gift of eternal happiness," and the modern cancer patient who commits suicide because he cannot bear that "his" cancer is killing him against his will, a hundred different attitudes are possible.

ILLNESS AS A REVERSIBLE STATE

We have seen, in a schematic fashion, that illness is an anomalous state of life for whomever comes to suffer it and participate in it. It is a process occurring over time and is therefore always changing. But illness is not only an anomalous state; it is also a correctable disorder in whose treatment the patient's person plays some part. Let us see, then, how an individual accomplishes this in his condition as a sick person. In order to clarify, it is necessary to distinguish three principal kinds of conduct: conduct in respect to himself, his doctor, and society.

The Sick Person vis-à-vis Himself

By deliberate exercise of his freedom, or by following subconscious tendencies, the sick person may desire his cure or not desire it. Scrutinizing this dual possibility is of the greatest importance for deciding what it means to be a good patient. Is the will to be cured a moral duty? In Western society, possible answers have been provided by the Greek, Christian, and secular traditions.

The Greek tradition. In ancient Greece it was believed that man springs from nature, and that nature itself tends toward the healing of illness, since health is a part of nature's good order. Further, the prime rule of morality for the Greek was conduct "in accordance with nature" (*kata physin*), because nature itself is "the divine." Thus, the sick person's wish to be cured was necessarily a serious and ineluctable moral duty. The entire *Corpus Hippocraticum* is saturated with this fundamental moral conviction. (An exception to this was when sovereign nature mysteriously decreed a patient's death *kat anakên*, through inexorable, fatal necessity.)

The Christian tradition. With the spread of Christianity, the root of the problem changed. If, in man's reality, there is something, "spirit," "person," that ontologically sees itself as higher than cosmic nature, and if the supreme realization of human destiny (life and eternal good) has a formally supernatural character, respect for the tendencies of nature cannot be an indisputable moral imperative for man. As a result, the will to be cured may or may not be a moral duty, according to the importance that Christianity attributes to the "natural order" of the cosmos, as the Greeks had been taught to understand it. Christians such as Taciano the Assyrian and Tertullian, because of their hostility toward the pagan world, opposed the adoption of the art of curing from the Greeks and proposed the inactive surrender of the sick person to the charity of his fellow men and to divine mercy. At the height of the Middle Ages, St. Bernard did not permit his monks any medication other than the "humble herbs" of the countryside. To seek a doctor's help seemed to him to be contrary to the purity of his order. A letter written by Ignatius Loyola shows the change that had occurred in ascetic Christianity after the Middle Ages. "I greatly desire that your Majesty impress upon your soul that it, like your body, belongs to your creator and Lord, who keeps good account of all things, and thus does not abandon unto weakness bodily nature, lest by its being weak, what is inward be unable to perform its function ... thus we ought to love and care for the body, inasmuch as it serves and assists the soul." Later, Ignatius wrote to Sister Theresa Rajadell, "With a healthy body, you will be able to do a great deal; with it sick, I don't know what you can do."

Even though the modern mind has made progress in understanding the phenomenal world, and even though man may be in this world only to fulfill his personal life and religious destiny, proper attention to oneself and to the medical care of the sick continues to be a clear moral duty. Such an attitude gained increasing force in the centuries after the Renaissance, and today no Christian would fail to subscribe to the moral rules regarding conduct in the face of pain (and thus sickness) which theologian Hans Küng proposes: "Do not look for pain, but endure it. Not only endure pain, but fight it. Not only fight pain, but transform it." Transform it, when it is inevitable, into the highest spiritual life.

The secular tradition. The progressive secularization of life in the West since the seventeenth century has added a new stance toward the problem of the will to be cured. Radically secularized man does not accept duties externally imposed by a being who is alien to the human condition and superior to it. For man, only autonomy informs morality and duty. Whatever the philosophy a man may use to understand his own reality, at the same time he believes that mind and freedom offer an operative principle to which the orderings of the cosmic world are subordinate. Otherwise, there could not be modern science or technology. Because of this, he believes himself to possess total ethical independence with respect to nature's laws and tendencies.

To the man fully human and humanly free belongs the right to his own death. The will to be cured could not be an absolute value for him; rather, the deliberate renunciation of treatment, euthanasia, and even suicide appear to him to be inalienable rights. In short, when secular man falls ill, his conscience feels completely free to want or not want to be cured (which, as the experience of sensitive doctors teaches, in no way excludes the subconscious existence of tendencies contrary to those occurring consciously).

Viewing the psychosocial situation from the perspective of a Kantian religious morality, Weizseaker (1951) has proposed that in the final analysis, the will to be cured is a categorical imperative for modern secular man. In other words, the moral decision to be cured is actually inherent and compelling. In the medical anthropology of Weizseaker, sickness is a "non-truth" of the sick person's existence, a state that alters the fully authentic realization of that existence (and, therefore, its truth). The patient, then, has within himself (and not because it is imposed from outside) the duty to reconquer with his health the essential and profound truth of his existence. If his illness becomes chronic and incurable, his duty is to achieve the greatest part of the truth possible for him—the "least harm," as Spanish Renaissance doctor Alfonso Chirino would say. If desperation does not unsettle his thinking, any sick person would be able to acknowledge this conception of his duty.

Conduct of the Sick Person *vis-à-vis* His Doctor

It is obvious that the strength of the desire to be cured is the basic determinant of the attitude the patient adopts with his doctor. In his analysis of the social role of the sick person in developed societies, Talcott Parsons (1951, 1972) has described the "institutional expectations" to which patients are subjected, the rules of conduct that society expects them to follow in order to be considered "normal" patients. For example, the sick person is expected to want to get well; to seek out medical advice; and, in the service of his own health, to cooperate with the doctor who attends him. Thus, from a developed society's point of view, whoever lacks the will to be cured, fails to seek out medical advice, and fails to actively and loyally cooperate with his doctor, cannot be considered a good patient.

The desire to cooperate with one's doctor may vary considerably according to one's social group. Within Western societies, this desire, and the feeling of moral duty from which it emanates, will be more frequent in better adjusted social groups, that is, ones in which the social integration of the individual is more disciplined. But not everything can be reduced to this simple rule, for the social judgment of what truly constitutes illness may vary among groups that at first glance appear to be identical. Further, the patient's changing disposition in the face of the medical assistance offered and his varying experiences with the doctor he has selected (or that society has imposed) give rise to conduct that may or may not fulfill Parsons's scheme. For example, society's acceptance of neurosis as a real illness is recent, and only in certain cultural circles has it taken hold fully. The medical-sociological studies of Hollingshead and Redlich (1953, 1958) have shown that in several New Haven social strata, suffering from a neurotic illness does not release one from social obligations, and that in such cases the neurotic is often considered responsible for his disorder. Numerous German authors (Deneke 1957; Huebschman 1959; Muller 1960; Mitscherlich 1960; Wagner 1960) have pointed out that the sick person's role in the *Krankenkassen* (health insurance plan) has been turned upside down: from once feeling indebted to his doctor, the patient has come to feel like a creditor, with a consequent change in his willingness to cooperate with his doctor. In the United States, Thomas Szasz (1958) has studied changes that have recently occurred in the social role of the sick person with respect to his doctor, particularly his psychiatrist. As we can see, the theme is a matter of great current concern and is very complex.

Conduct of the Sick Person vis-à-vis Society

If sickness is a reversible disorder, the sick person ought to desire his cure and actively and sincerely cooperate toward it for purely social reasons (even when he may be able to give these reasons an underlying religious or philosophical justification). Several of the institutional expectations that Parsons has assigned to the social role of the patient are based on this duty. Such reasons are diverse: the sick person may spread his illness to those around him; health is an important precondition for an individual's participation in the social order;

sickness causes a moral affliction in those who look on the patient with love or compassion; illness frequently disturbs the economy of the social group to which one and others belong. There is no doubt that, by finding himself attached to a society, the sick person has a duty to cooperate willingly in the technical care of his ailment. But are the social mores which demand the fulfillment of this ethical norm possessed by all individuals and social groups in equal measure? Undoubtedly not. Similarly, there can be good patients and bad patients for reasons of strictly social character. Even a cursory look at the studies of medical sociology that examine the roles and attitudes of the sick will demonstrate this phenomenon (Freeman, Levine, and Reeder 1963; Coe 1970; Jaco 1972).

THE GOOD PATIENT

We have discussed the two principal modes of conduct of the sick person in the face of illness: understanding illness as an anomalous state and seeing it as a correctable disorder. Thus, we can now ask about the conditions in which a sick person becomes a good patient with respect to himself, his doctor, and the society.

The Sick Person vis-à-vis Himself

Aware of his own illness, and reacting to it, a sick person can be considered a good patient when his conduct conforms to the following norms:

1. When there is an attitude of active acceptance of the illness. Impatient or desperate rebellion, or excessive resignation before the vicissitude of suffering are not the responses of the good patient.
2. When the sick person sees illness as a chance occurrence, susceptible to elimination through intelligence and technique or as a test by which one may gain merit or worth. However, the patient should take no excessive self-satisfaction in the subtle eminence that being sick may bring with it. In present society, the interpretation of illness as a punishment is an obstacle to being a good patient.
3. When there is minimal participation by the sick person in the genesis and configuration of his illness, though he remains author and actor in it.
4. When the sick person makes the illness his own and takes possession of it in such a way that the "my" by which possession is expressed ("my" ulcer, "my" mitral stenosis) does not go beyond an interim "ownership," and does not indicate some deep-seated intent to use it to manipulate others.
5. When the sick person has the will to be cured, even though unconscious tendencies may oppose it (tendencies which, when they exist, should be discovered by the doctor and methodically eliminated).

6. When the sick person is aware that because he is sick, he really needs more than he would deserve in the normal course of things. Man can live in this respect according to the contrasting models of Narcissus and Pygmalion. The beautiful Narcissus sees his figure in the water's reflection, admires himself, and thinks, "I deserve everything I need." The sculptor Pygmalion falls in love with the figure of a woman he himself has carved, vehemently wishes the statue transformed into a woman of flesh and blood, and recognizes with humility that he has neither the power nor the merit for such a deed. As a result he thinks, "I need more than I deserve." Only by acting according to this second model can the sick person be a good patient.

The Sick Person vis-à-vis His Doctor

To be a good patient from this second perspective, the fulfillment of the following norms is necessary:

1. The sick person is reasonably obedient, but not absolutely submissive. By obeying his doctor, the sick person should not cease to be a free human being, a person. A slave's obedience is not the best kind for being a good patient in times of illness. Utilizing Reisman's terminology, one could say that the good patient is found in the center of the space that separates the other-directed man from the inner-directed man.
2. The sick person opens himself truthfully to his physician. Whether his confidence in whomever treats him is great or small, the sick person owes his doctor the truth about himself as soon as the doctor asks. Even when he confides little in his physician, the sick person can and ought to be a good patient.
3. The sick person abstains from self-medication, or at least, exercises great prudence with it. In order to be a good patient, as the ancient Hippocratics knew, the sick person ought to know something about his illness, according to his intelligence and his upbringing. With regard to self-medication, it is only by acting prudently in the light of this knowledge that the sick person can be a good patient.

The Sick Person vis-à-vis Society

A good patient must fulfill the following social duties in the face of his illness:

1. To the extent that it is possible for him, not spreading his disease. Therefore, diligent cooperation in the determination that his illness, if it is contagious, not affect others, is expected of him.
2. Careful avoidance of the problems that his illness can produce in those around him.

3. The effective desire to actively reintegrate into his social group as soon as possible.
4. Reduction to a minimum of the economic demands and burdens that illness brings with it.
5. If he belongs to a wealthy society, clear awareness of the many sick people who are suffering but cannot be cared for as he has been.

THE DOCTOR AND THE GOOD PATIENT

There is one important final question: How many sick people can be good patients? In principle, all of them can. It is certainly true that underlying circumstances (personal character or the social or cultural group delivering medical care, for example) can increase the possibility that a sick person may be a bad patient. But the best evidence that a doctor is a good doctor—which means that he or she has both technical competence and the will to help—is the fact that all of his or her patients somehow turn out to be good patients. It does not seem unfair to say to a doctor, as a kind of qualifying test, "Tell me how many good patients you have, and I will tell you how good a doctor you are."

Bibliography

Bernbeu, E. 1958. "The Effects of Severe Crippling on the Development of a Group of Children." *Psychiatry* 21: 169-94.

Blum, R.H. 1956. *Physician-Patient Relationship.* San Francisco: California Medical Association.

Blum, R.H., Sadusk, J., and Waterson, R. 1960. *The Management of the Doctor-Patient Relationship.* New York: McGraw-Hill.

Coe, R.M. 1970. *Sociology of Medicine.* New York: McGraw-Hill.

Deneke, J.F.V. 1957. *Gesundheitspolitik.* Stuttgart: McGraw-Hill.

Feifel, H. 1959. *The Meaning of Death.* New York: McGraw-Hill.

Freeman, H.E., Levine, S., and Reeder, L.G. 1963. *Handbook of Medical Sociology.* Englewood Cliffs, NJ: Prentice-Hall.

Gomez Bosque, P. 1960. "Topología de la Intimidad. Los Fundamentos Ontológicos y Morfo-funcionales de las Relaciones Psico-somáticas." *Actas Luso-Espanolas de Neurología y Psiquiatría* 19: 149-93.

Haefner, H. 1963. "Psychosomatische Medizin und Leibphänomenologie." In *Werden und Handeln.* Stuttgart: Hippokdrates-Verlag.

Hollingshead, A.B., and Redlich, F.C. 1953. "Social Class and Psychiatric Disorders." *American Sociological Review* 18: 163-69.

_____ . 1958. *Social Class and Mental Illness: A Community Study.* New York: John Wiley and Sons.

Huebschman, H. 1957. "Der Artz und die soziale Wirklichkeit." *Frankfurter Hefte* 12: 573-80.

Jaco, E.G., ed. 1972. *Patients, Physicians and Illness: A Sourcebook in Behavioral Science and Health.* 2d ed. New York: Free Press.

Laín Entralgo, P. 1960. "Enfermedad y Vida Humana." In *Ocio y trabajo.* Madrid.

_____ . 1961. *Enfermedad y Pecado.* Barcelona.

_____ . 1964. *La Relacíon Medico-Enfermo.* Madrid.

_____ . 1968. *El Estado de Enfermedad.* Madrid.

_____ . 1970. *La medicina hipocratica.* Madrid.

Mitscherlich, A. 1960. "Der genormte Patient." *Bundesarbeitsblatt* 11: 402-18.

Muller, A. 1960. "Subjektive Aspekte der Krankenversicherungs-Neuregelung." *Bundersarbeitsblatt* 11: 394-406.

Parsons, T. 1951. *The Social System.* Glencoe, IL: Free Press.

———. 1972. "Definitions of Health and Illness in the Light of American Values and Social Structure." In *Patients, Physicians and Illness: A Sourcebook in Behavioral Science and Health,* edited by E.G. Jaco. 2d ed. New York: Free Press.

Rof Carballo, J. 1952. *Cerebro Interno y Mundo Emocional.* Barcelona.

———. 1960. *Urdimbre Afectiva y Enfermedad.* Barcelona.

Schaefer, H. 1960. "Der Patient, seine Krankheit und der Artz." *Bundesarbeitsblatt* 11: 402-21.

Spitz, R. 1945. "Hospitalism." In *Psychoanalytic Study of the Child,* edited by Ruth S. Eissler et al. New York: International Universities Press.

Szasz, T.S. 1958. "Scientific Method and Social Role in Medicine and Psychiatry." *Archives of Internal Medicine* 101: 228-38.

Uexkull, Th. von. 1951. "Das Problem der Befindenwisen und seine Bedektung für eine medizinische Phänomenologie." *Psyche* 5: 401-32.

Wagner, K. 1960. "Kassenpatient und Kassenarzt in der Gegenwart." *Bundesarbeitsblatt* 11: 403-10.

Weizseaker, V. von. 1951. *Der kranke Mensch.* Stuttgart: K.F. Koehler.

Zborowski, M. 1952. "Cultural Components in Response to Pain." *Journal of Social Issues* 8: 16-30.

Rights and Responsibilities of Patients:
A Commentary on Pedro Laín Entralgo

James F. Childress

It is a great honor for me to comment on the paper by Pedro Laín Entralgo, whose work I have long admired. In view of the themes of this volume, I wish to focus on the place of the person in Professor Laín Entralgo's description of the "good patient." The basic thrust of my argument will be that the person has a secondary or subsidiary place in Laín Entralgo's understanding of the good patient. Before I develop this argument, however, some preliminary observations are in order.

First, Eric Cassell has contended that this volume is designed to get beyond biomedical ethics. This contention is ambiguous. It may mean that our task is to examine a range of questions that have nothing to do with biomedical ethics, or, alternatively, that our test is to consider some questions that are presupposed by biomedical ethics. The latter interpretation is more plausible. Insofar as conceptions of the person in medicine are presupposed by biomedical ethics, it is therefore important to consider their implications for biomedical ethics. Indeed, it may even be possible and necessary to test various conceptions of the person in medicine by what they imply for ethical judgments in medicine.

A second preliminary observation is that cultural perspectives can shape the ways in which problems are formulated. During a recent trip to China to study the interrelations of ethics, public policy, and health care, participants in our group frequently asked Chinese philosophers, physicians, scientists, and policy makers how they handled some of our important problems. Often the response was: "That's not a problem here." In my comments on Professor Laín Entralgo's paper, I am aware that significant cultural differences may shape our different perceptions and formulations of the problems.

Not only should we analyze and understand such differences, but we should also trace their implications for medicine and health care. Only then can we consider their adequacy or inadequacy.

ANALYSIS OF PROFESSOR LAÍN ENTRALGO'S ARGUMENT

Professor Laín Entralgo's thesis is that "the good patient is the person who, as a patient, fully and completely fulfills his essential being" (1985, p. 128). He considers two different perspectives on the state of being a patient. The first perspective focuses on the patient as a person, while the second focuses on patienthood as a correctable deficiency or reversible condition. He maintains that the former is subordinate to the latter.

The first perspective includes the patient's generic feelings and especially "how the sick person conducts himself in the face of his illness" (p. 130). In particular, Professor Laín Entralgo analyzes the person's affective and interpretive responses to illness as an anomaly. He offers an excellent portrayal of a range of these responses and then considers the person's role in his own illness.

But this first perspective—the patient's involvement in and response to illness—merely provides "valuable and important elements for defining what precisely constitutes a good patient" (p. 133). Which elements mark the good patient and which the bad one? Professor Laín Entralgo's answer depends almost exclusively on the second perspective on being a patient: the condition of patienthood considered as a "correctable deficiency," a "reversible state," "in whose treatment the patient's person plays some part." The part played by the patient's person is, I would suggest, almost instrumental. The patient's person becomes a means or mechanism for correcting this deficiency. The emphasis is not on the person who has his own life plans, projects, and commitments, but on the person who can help to correct the deficiency of patienthood by certain attitudes, dispositions, and actions toward himself, his doctors, and his society.

These attitudes, dispositions, and actions all derive from the patient's religious, moral, and social *duty* to will to be cured. To cite one example, Professor Laín Entralgo rejects the modern, secular concept of autonomy which appears to allow people to refuse medical treatment and even to commit suicide when they do not want to be cured or when life does not appear to them to be worth living. Following Weizseaker, Professor Laín Entralgo insists that the will to be cured is a categorical imperative for modern man: "If desperation does not unsettle his thinking, any sick person would be able to acknowledge this conception of his duty" (p. 137). This duty to will to be cured becomes Laín Entralgo's fundamental criterion for selecting the affective and interpretive responses that mark the good patient. Thus, the appropriate affective response is "active acceptance," and the appropriate interpretive response is "chance" or "test." These responses are "good" because they enable the patient to discharge his duty to will to be cured. Likewise, the good doctor is one who can induce the patient to be a good patient.

SOME CRITICAL QUESTIONS

Several aspects of Professor Laín Entralgo's interpretation of the good patient appear to be problematic. At the very least, they indicate points of tension between his position and a position that emphasizes that the patient as a person has his own life plans, values, and the right of autonomy (e.g., the right to refuse treatment).

First, *good* need not always be used as a morally evaluative term. It has many nonmoral evaluative uses as well, for example, "that is a good car." Professor Laín Entralgo, however, conflates *good* with *morally good*, at least in his evaluation of patients. Of course, his good patient may not be morally good in a total or holistic sense. But he is morally good insofar as his affective and interpretive responses enable him to discharge his moral duties as a patient. The moral duty to will recovery or cure implies other moral duties, such as willing cooperation with doctors in technical care. While it is possible that the social reasons to will to be cured are sufficient, Professor Laín Entralgo emphasizes and builds on the moral reason.

Second, the language of *rights* is either overlooked or rejected in this characterization of the good patient. It is unclear whether the good patient recognizes no rights or willingly relinquishes them. In either case, the patient's *duties* and *needs*, rather than his rights, are dominant. For example, the good patient is aware that because he is sick, he really needs more than he *deserves*. It is possible that Professor Laín Entralgo may only oppose the assertion of a positive right to health care, but what he says may also apply to other rights within health care (e.g., autonomy).

Surely the language of rights is overused and overextended in the United States. We frequently appear to suppose that there are no significant moral arguments apart from the language of rights. But even so, an interpretation of the good patient that does not include the patient's rights may be deficient. The language of rights arms the patient. It makes the patient an agent who controls one end of the chain of rights and obligations connecting patients and physicians. In a pluralistic society beset with major value disputes, the patient's right of autonomy is particularly important, for it limits the professional's or the society's control over the patient even when the control is held to be beneficial to the patient.

Third, because of its emphasis on the patient's duties and needs, rather than his rights, Professor Laín Entralgo's model of the physician-patient relationship appears to be paternalistic (or parentalistic). There are many different models of the physician-patient relationship, some descriptive, some normative, and some mixed. These models draw on other human relationships in order to illuminate the relationships between health care professionals and patients. In the several models that focus on agency and values in the process of decision making in medicine and health care, the physician's role (or the physician) has been characterized as (1) paternalist, (2) technician, (3) contractor, (4) partner, (5) friend, and (6) bureaucrat.

In his book *Doctor and Patient* (1969), Professor Laín Entralgo stresses that the medical relationship is not only comradeship or partnership, but also friendship, because "man is an individual and his illness a state affecting his personality" (p. 197). The doctor's "friendship for the patient should consist above all in a desire to give effective technical help—benevolence conceived and realized in technical terms" (p. 242). But as Professor Laín Entralgo's present paper makes clear, decision making within this friendship is not symmetrical. Indeed, in terms of decision making, the model can best be characterized as paternalistic; paternalism at least appears to be an implication of the qualities of the good patient. A health care professional may choose to reject or to acquiesce in a patient's wishes, choices, and actions for the patient's own good—the patient's needs and duties. Benevolence may override autonomy, which, in any event, is not identified as a right.

In a very different model, the principle of autonomy, or respect for autonomy (self-rule or self-determination), requires respect for the patient as a person who can competently and freely choose (or acknowledge) and act on his own values. Some commentators hold that the person's autonomy is the goal of medicine, but autonomy is also important as a limit or constraint and not merely as a goal. Of course, autonomy can be justifiably overridden in order to protect others (e.g., from infectious diseases). More controversial are violations of autonomy solely to protect the patient himself, because these appear to offer an affront, an insult, and an indignity to the person. They treat an adult person as a child, that is, as one who cannot take responsibility for his own welfare. They fail to respect the patient-person as an equal.

Professor Laín Entralgo implies that certain life plans make a bad patient because they interfere with the duty to will to be cured, for example, if a patient refuses curative treatment because he interprets the disease as punishment and passively submits (or even actively rebels). Paternalism toward such patients may be either weak or strong

(Feinberg 1973, pp. 50-51). Strong paternalism would override even the competent patient's free and informed wishes, choices, and actions. Weak paternalism, however, would override a patient's express will only when there is good reason to think that the patient is not able to exercise his autonomy because of some defect or limitation. Professor Laín Entralgo appears to acknowledge strong paternalism, but only under the guise of weak paternalism. That is, if the patient does not will to be cured (perhaps because his pain and suffering are great), he violates a moral duty; he would acknowledge (and presumably act on) that duty if his mind were not unsettled by desperation.

Fourth, an implication of the three preceding points is that Professor Laín Entralgo's paternalism is moralistic because of the moral duty to will to be cured. This moralism is evident in the claim that for a person to be a good patient he should have had only "minimal participation" in the genesis of his illness. But it is not clear why a person who has brought about his own illness, either through subconscious factors or through voluntary risk-taking (e.g., a cigarette smoker who gets lung cancer), cannot be a good patient. Perhaps Professor Laín Entralgo assumes the primacy of the value of health, and a duty to preserve it, prior to the medical relationship. Other life plans and risk budgets (Fried 1970, part III) that subordinate health to other values appear to be rejected on moralistic grounds. Personal autonomy is qualified by a moral and social duty to will to be cured and to stay well. Within medicine itself, there appears to be a single legitimate goal; other ends, goals, and values that patients as persons want to realize through medicine appear to be regarded as inappropriate.

Fifth, perhaps it would be better to substitute another term for *good* in describing and evaluating patients. Other terms might enable us to capture more clearly the importance of the patient's own values and projects and his rights, as well as his duties. One possible term, more widely used in theological than in philosophical circles, is *responsible*. Two authors who use the term *responsible patient*, rather than *good patient*, contend that it is difficult to be a responsible patient largely because of the success of preventive and curative medicine (Siegler and Osmond 1979). One consequence of this success is that we have limited experience with patienthood, as well as unrealistic expectations of health and medicine; thus, it is difficult to play the role of patient responsibly, that is, with due attention to rights and to duties.

Bibliography

Feinberg, J. 1973. *Social Philosophy*. Englewood Cliffs, NJ: Prentice-Hall.

Fried, C. 1970. *An Anatomy of Values*. Cambridge, MA: Harvard University Press.

Laín Entralgo, P. 1969. *Doctor and Patient*. Translated by F. Partridge. New York: McGraw-Hill.

_____ . 1985. "What Does the Word *Good* Mean in *Good Patient?*", pp. 127-143 in this volume.

Siegler, M., and Osmond, H. 1979. *Patienthood: The Art of Being a Responsible Patient*. New York: Macmillan.

Uses of the Subjective in Medical Practice

Eric J. Cassell

WHY TACKLE THE SUBJECTIVE IN MEDICAL PRACTICE?

Critics of current medical practice, pointing to its depersonalization, often imply that merely limiting the place of science and technology in medicine would somehow direct medical care toward those needs of patients that are not yet fulfilled. I do not believe that placing restraints on science and technology will solve medicine's deficiencies. Instead, the scientific tools of the physician should be brought to bear in new ways and on new problems. In particular, medicine must shift away from an exclusive focus on disease toward a primary concern for the sick person, and there are signs that this has already begun. This shift does not portend a diminishing of science, but rather a larger understanding of what is meant by science.

As in the best of our past, the sick themselves will show us the way. In the late eighteenth and early nineteenth centuries, for example, it was a return to clinical realities that brought an end to theorizing about the nature of disease (and Nature herself) and formed the basis for modern concepts of disease. And it was those new ideas about disease, firmly rooted in clinical medicine, that enabled scientific methods to be focused on the problems of the sick. We are justly proud of our system of medical education, but the aspect of education in which we take the greatest pride—bedside education—is becoming progressively less patient-oriented. Today, many students look past the patients to get at their diseases, studying the results of laboratory and x-ray examinations more often than they examine their patients. In all of this, the subjective aspects of illness—what patients say, desire, think, fear, feel, and care about, and how and why they behave the way they do toward disease, doctors, symptoms, their bodies, themselves, and others—seem to be an impediment to staying at the bedside and to understanding sickness. These particular and individual

151

concerns of the patient are taken to be an obstruction, as one of my students said, "that stands between me and what I really know about, which is disease."

Perhaps the greatest advantage of scientific methods and technology is their objectivity; they are all rooted in the measurable, the calculable. Conversely, supposedly the greatest obstacle to attending to the larger human dimensions of sickness is their "subjectivity." Or, to put it another way, when we say that the patient's report was subjective, we imply that a different patient might have reported differently about the same thing. What is it about subjectivity that makes these differences, and why are they important for doctors? In an important sense it is our lack of understanding of the subjective—those aspects of illness that are shaped by the patient's mental life—that has driven us from the bedside and that keeps us from utilizing to the fullest capacity the skills we possess.

There seems no choice but to attack the problem of the subjective. We have made enormous strides towards an objective knowledge of the body and there is more to come, but if we are to return to the bedside we simply must give greater credence to the patient's subjective life. We will not be able to do this, however, unless and until the various meanings that have become attached to the terms *subjective* or *subjectivity* in medical practice are sufficiently understood so that they can be worked with on a day-to-day basis.

Whose Subjectivity Are We Talking About?

Discussions of subjective information in medical care usually make no distinction between the subjectivity of the physician and that of the patient. In this paper, unless I specify otherwise, I am speaking of the patient's subjectivity. The distinction is vital: what the physician knows of the patient's needs, desires, feelings, body sensations, reported symptoms, remembrances, understandings, and so on is not subjective knowledge. Instead, it is information that can be part of the objective knowledge of the physician. The physician knows those things about patients in the same way that he or she knows that patients who have a certain cast to their faces or pick at the bedclothes are very sick. This knowledge is as objective as the knowledge that certain bacteria on a slide are pneumococci. Those things are part of the objective knowledge of physicians even though they are not susceptible to numerical measurement. Like virtually all knowledge, it is probabilistic, that is, it is true only within certain limits. But accuracy and objectivity are not coextensive even though they are often confused.

The word *objective* is frequently used in the following sense: "Nine of thirty-five patients ... had a new episode of venous thromboembolism that was confirmed by objective tests." In this context *objective* means that the tests used were able to detect thromboembolism without reliance on the patients' reports. Further, it also indicates that the test results, numerical values, scans, and so forth will be available for review by other observers, and thus are potentially free of the physician's subjective bias. This elimination of the possible subjective bias of both patient and physician seems to offer a great advantage. But a measure of disease is not necessarily better simply because it is objective in those two senses. The recent literature on exercise testing for coronary artery disease, for example, indicates that both the specificity and sensitivity of that objective measure of disease is greatly increased if the patient reports typical angina pectoris. These studies suggest that the history of the disease—the patient's subjective report—has greater accuracy then the objective test alone.

For medical practice, such standards as accuracy, precision, sensitivity, and specificity are related primarily to methodology. It is true that the methods physicians use to extract all of the information contained in patients' subjective reports lack the precision of other techniques; they do not approach the richness, complexity, or subtlety of the patients' subjective lives and may be interfered with by the patient's own thought processes. But these drawbacks do not make the information acquired less a part of the physician's objective knowledge or less vital to medical practice. In this context, we should remember that the first stethoscopes—wooden cylinders with a hole bored through them—were primitive, but nonetheless effective. They supplied a kind of information not otherwise available.

Some Meanings of the Subjective Put Aside in This Paper

Dealing with subjectivity is particularly difficult, in part because it has so many different philosophical connotations. However, some understanding of the concept of the subjective can be arrived at that will serve as a basis for its use in medical practice. Let me begin by indicating two senses of the word *subjective* that I will not address. In the first sense of the word, *subjective* refers to relative perception: you see a red tie and I see a red tie; how do we know that we both see the same thing? You hear a heart murmur and I hear a heart murmur; how do we know that we both heard the same thing? We do not. The wavelength of the red can be measured and reproduced, the sound of the heart murmur accurately and objectively described, but whether or not these perceptions are experienced in precisely the same way by both of us cannot be known. They are subjectively relative, unalterably idiosyncratic to the subject. The fact is, however, that we both can learn to respond in a similar manner to the same stimulus. Thus, at least in this context, the fact that stimuli are subjectively relative does not pose a large barrier to medical advancement.

The second sense of the word *subjective*—the inner state or body sensations of a subject—is very important in medicine. Indeed, it is what is most commonly referred to when physicians say that something is subjective. The patient says that something "hurts," that he or she "just does not feel right," that an arm feels "funny," that nausea or shortness of breath is present, and so on. Although these are unconfirmable symptoms, they are precisely the kind of statements that generally initiate the medical act. Notice that I did not include qualifiers with those symptoms. But I could have mentioned intermittent pain or brief pain, waves of nausea or steady nausea, without changing this sense of the subjective. Although those adjectives add qualifiers, the phrases describe basic symptoms, and I do not believe that raw symptom reports are our problem. However, had I said "terrible," "agonizing," or "silly" pain, or "pain like colitis," this sense of the subjective would have begun to change. Qualitative reports of body sensations like pain, nausea, or dyspnea are often unverifiable or verifiable only with difficulty and are, therefore, clearly subjective. However, despite the medical importance of such symptom reports, I do not believe they are the aspect of patients' subjectivity that is so troubling to medicine about subjectivity in general. For when a patient reports pain, nausea, dyspnea, and so on, it is overwhelmingly the case that those sensations exist in the patient's body. To believe otherwise is to believe that someone might feel a sensation where no sensation existed, which would be strange, or that the patient is simply lying, which is unusual. I am reminded of a Chinese patient in the Bellevue emergency room who spoke no English. I asked the interpreter to find out what was the matter. Soon the patient and interpreter were arguing loudly. I finally prevailed on the interpreter to tell me what the patient was saying. "He says his chest splashes when he steps off the curb, but he's crazy." Of course, he was neither lying nor crazy, and his chest x-ray confirmed hydropneumothorax. What patients report is overwhelmingly the truth.

THE SUBJECTIVE AS PERSONAL MEANING

What is there about adding words like *terrible, silly, frightening,* or ... *like colitis* that changes the dimension of subjectivity, of human consciousness, into which such symptom reports fall? Such adjectives add a kind of meaning. And the moment that kind of meaning is present, we are dealing with the area of the subjective that is as absolutely vital to medical practice as it is confusing and misunderstood. Prior to adding words like *agonizing* or ... *like colitis*, the patient was merely transmitting information about physical sensations. Since this is a kind of information that only the subject, the person experiencing it, can know, we call it subjective information. Much information with relevance to medicine can be known almost exclusively to the person who experiences it. But this becomes more than simply information about physical sensations when meaning is added by the process of interpretation. Meaning itself is a difficult issue because so many senses of the term exist. Two are particularly useful in the context of medical care.

Meaning as Significance

On one level, to mean is to signify, to imply. Dark clouds signify rain; high left ventricular end-diastolic pressure implies a fall in left ventricular output. Those are meanings of dark clouds and left ventricular end-diastolic pressure, respectively. Physicians constantly use that sense of *meaning* as they work out a chain of explanation of physiologic events. This sense of meaning is often expressed by the phrase, "the consequences of...." The similarity between this sense of meaning and the term *objective* is quickly apparent. Those physiologic processes go on in bodies, and it does not matter whose body it is. The knee bone is connected to the thigh bone, and the thigh bone is connected to the hip bone, and that is just the fact of the matter.

Meaning as Personal Importance

The other sense of *meaning* is conveyed by saying that we know what something "means" when we know how important it is. Asked whether a fact is important or not, it would be natural to ask "important to whom?" This use of *meaning* always implies that there is a person for whom something does or does not have meaning. In this sense, dark clouds mean that tomorrow's picnic will be ruined, and an elevated left ventricular end-diastolic pressure means that the patient with the recent myocardial infarction has a bad prognosis—sadness will soon follow. This sense of meaning introduces and entails a measure of particularity. For example, if two patients have fever, chest pain, and cough, those events signify pneumonia for both of them. But suppose that one patient lost both parents and his two siblings from pneumonia, while the other had never encountered the illness. The meaning of pneumonia to those two patients is vastly different, although the diagnostic implications of the symptoms are the same. For one, however, dread and threat to life are part of the meaning of pneumonia, overtones that are absent from the conception of the other patient. Thus, meaning of this second kind is inevitably personal meaning. The importance of the facts is personal and individual.

It is this area of subjectivity, which encompasses the particular significance and personal importance of things, that I believe must be confronted by medicine if we are to remain directed to our mission of caring for the sick. This sense of the subjective, as personal meanings, is vital to effective diagnosis and treatment. In proposing the reincorporation of personal meanings in medical practice, it may seem that I am suggesting a return to the anecdotal in medicine, unsupported by evidence as a basis for action. Alternatively it may appear that I am suggesting the substitution of value judgments, intuitions, or professional authority for objective evidence. Although the direction I am suggesting carries that danger, that is most definitely not what I mean. My proposal can be clarified by looking briefly at the morass that existed in medicine before science began to clarify human biology in a way that made rational medicine possible.

Medical science and the therapeutic effectiveness of physicians could not have progressed to their present state without the development of objective experimental methods. Much of the difficulty in research methodology, in the laboratory as well as in controlled clinical trials, comes from the need to eliminate human bias, institutional or individual. This is to prevent the distortion of any findings by the particular beliefs or values of the investigator. *Beliefs* is another word for the "significance" aspect of personal meaning, and *values* is another word for "importance to a particular person." Thus the phrase, "beliefs and the values attached to them" is coextensive with "personal meaning." Medicine could not, therefore, have progressed had it not been possible to develop scientific methods unbiased by the personal meanings of investigators.

It may seem paradoxical to suggest that progress in medical care, and even in research, requires not further freedom from value contamination but rather the intensive pursuit and systematization of the valuing subject. Whether a research method can be entirely value-free or objective may be open to debate; but a value-free human medicine, a medicine free of meaning to the subject is impossible— it is, in fact, a contradiction in terms.

MEDICAL CARE IS INHERENTLY CONCERNED WITH VALUE

Physicians take for granted that preventing premature death, extending meaningful life, improving the quality of life, and diminishing unnecessary pain and suffering are fundamental parts of their job. Those goals are tied to individual values and beliefs; they are important to people, both physicians and patients. The meaning of *premature death, meaningful life, pain, quality of life,* and *suffering,* for example, differ in important ways from one person to another.

Given the nature of the medical profession, no alternative primary goals are possible, goals that are objective and free of human value. Confusion often arises on this point because there certainly are goals of treatment that can be measured objectively, but it is usually forgotten that these are always in the service of, subsidiary to, some value-laden goal. For instance, arthritis may cause painful suffering and when it does there will usually be a decreased range of joint motion. Thus, one can objectively measure an improvement in the range of motion in a joint that would suggest, but not be the same as, a reduction in suffering or a better quality of life. The measurement of blood pressure is also objective, but it has utility in the care of patients only because, for example, the disease hypertension can diminish the quality of life and cause suffering or premature death—which are irreducibly value-laden or subjective issues. Objective facts, therefore, are important to practicing physicians and effectively serve to guide their actions in large part because these facts are tied to personal meanings. Those objective facts also signify physiologic events quite apart from their subjective importance. But, in that sense, the falling blood pressure is no more important than a leaf falling in a forest.

Medical practice is ineluctably subjective, subordinate to the human values and personal meaning of both physicians and patients. That may have been obscured in our recent history for two reasons. The first is that the meanings and values to which medicine is dedicated are virtually universal. They are sufficiently common to all sick persons in the Western medical tradition so that they tend to disappear from conscious view, becoming invisible features of the background against which other aspects of medicine are viewed. Such universal values reappear in rituals and symbols, for example, the oaths read at medical school graduations or the picture of the Good Samaritan which is the logo of The New York Hospital. Another more important reason might be that the problems and pitfalls of subjectivity were enlarged out of proportion and its importance obscured as the subjective became the target in the battles of the last century to create an objective science of medicine. The realization that there is an objective world and that a science of human biology is possible have been hard won. Those goals of science had to be wrestled free from things that may be associated with subjectivity, such as magic, superstition, religion, personal authority, beliefs in special powers, and so on. Thus, during the fight to achieve a scientific medicine, subjectivity has been seen as the enemy while, paradoxically, the inherently personal, value-laden goals of medicine remained, often below awareness. Now the effort must be continued in a different direction as human values and intentionality become critically important.

Objectivity and science have become so essential to medical practice and thinking that I do not believe we will return to prescientific medicine if a disciplined understanding of the personal is attempted. Indeed, if all the subjective meanings that underlie medical care were truly universal—as our creeds suggest but clinical practice denies— then, perhaps, no such systematic study of the subjective would be necessary. But while many of the human values underlying medical practice may indeed be universal, they are also sufficiently particular so that doctors and their skills cannot be allowed to focus on universals alone. If it is to be effective and not destructive, the science and technology of medicine must be directed to the particular needs of individual patients. We are all aware of the dangers inherent in the inappropriate use of advanced technology, such as drugs, tests, and procedures. Inappropriate use does not mean, generally, application to the wrong disease or pathophysiologic state but, rather, that they are not matched to the personal needs of a particular patient. Post-terminal resuscitative procedures are a case in point.

INDIVIDUALITY OF MEANINGS

The individuality of meanings requires special attention. The kind of personal meanings that are fundamental to medicine are neither uniformly universal nor idiosyncratically personal. For example, phrases such as "unnecessary suffering" and "quality of life" cannot be defined precisely, despite many efforts. They are metaphors that mean slightly different things to each of us and thus are not truly universal, but each of these meanings remains within the root meanings of the language. Without a common language—that is, if meanings were completely idiosyncratic—no communication between individuals would be possible. Further, language and personal meanings are neither appropriated entirely by individuals for their own use nor completely universal; they arise out of historical background, are derivative of culture and family, express themselves in a context, and are embedded in a matrix of other meanings. Because of those origins personal meaning is shared and knowable; it is accessible via questions, as well as to observations of lifestyle and behavior. These are the routes to knowledge that medicine must begin to investigate, not for their own sake (as in the social sciences) but for what they can contribute to the practice of medicine. To base medical action on the assumption that personal meanings are all shared, that what is meaningful to one person is identically meaningful to all, is to ignore the individuality of meanings. Such an assumption of shared meanings would be like saying that a well-trained physician who is dedicated and cares about his or her patient knows alone what is best for that patient. Those days of the "doctor knows best" mentality are, happily, over.

How Personal Meaning Functions

How do meanings function in medicine and what part do they play in the care of patients? In the simplest terms, people act because of the meanings they assign to those actions. For example, patients go to doctors because of what their symptoms mean to them, not because of the objective significance of the symptoms. Information constantly flows toward each individual. A pain is information, as is the doctor's behavior, a runny nose, the context of events, and virtually everything that a person perceives from the body, the unconscious, the outside world, and so on. But information must always be assigned a meaning; it must be given both significance and personal importance. Within the subjective life, those two things are inseparable. The significance of a fact is always interpreted within a network. And some networks are more important than others; for example, information that suggests danger to health is more important than other information. An actual example may illustrate the point.

A sixty-two-year-old woman was admitted to the hospital in the beginning of January with weight loss, hepatomegaly, and anemia. She had metastatic carcinoma to the liver from the colon. This quote is taken from her initial history: "So then I realized that I was losing weight, but not because I'm on a diet. Sometimes, I go on a diet because I'm heavy. I'm still heavy but I was glad I was losing it because I could stand it. Then I started to think to myself, 'But why am I losing it?' "

The doctor asked when she had started to think that way, and she replied, "About the end of December." It turned out that at a physical examination in November, the woman had been told of anemia and a twenty-pound weight loss, and she was advised to have some tests; these she put off until the end of December. Why did she wait so long and what finally made her act? She commented on the weight loss:

> It was nothing sudden; it was all a gradual thing. Maybe in weeks' time I felt, um—my dresses are getting a little loose on me. I wondered why and I realized it was my appetite; I was eating smaller meals. I was delighted because I was losing weight and that's what I wanted to do.
>
> But then I found that I would eat, like, meat, vegetables, and potatoes, and then I would be filled. And I had no desire for dessert. And I said to myself, "This is not me," because I always loved desserts.

Asked when she first realized it was not her, she said, "About Christmas."

This patient interpreted the information about her weight loss in two different networks with vastly different importance to her health. At first, the weight loss was given a positive meaning within the context of a lifelong battle with her weight. Why would she go to a doctor for that? A doctor might even interfere with her weight loss. But when the weight loss was coupled with the "that isn't me" fact of not wanting dessert, an ominous meaning was attached and she promptly sought medical advice.

Endless examples could be cited to illustrate how personal meaning determines behavior. Going to physicians, taking medication, being operated on, following a diet, and so on, are all behaviors. In fact, it would be difficult to find an example of behavior not related to meanings. It would also be difficult to find a disease in which the patient's behavior in regard to symptoms, disabilities, restrictions, treatment, and so forth, did not in some way affect the presentation, course, and outcome of the illness. It should also be obvious that the same event is assigned different meanings by different people and thus that behavior varies. We are all aware, just as in the example cited, that the same facts may be given very different meanings by the same individual—witness the health behavior of physicians.

WHY THE SUBJECTIVE HAS SURFACED NOW

Given the crucial role of personal meaning in medical practice, it is difficult to understand why its systematic study is not already a part of medicine. It cannot be that the subjective disappeared solely because universal meanings guide practice. There is certainly no universality about the perceived significance of weight loss, infections, surgery, diet, exercise, and so on. Rather, I believe that the subjective— personal meanings—has become increasingly important to medical care for two quite different reasons. The first, discussed in the Introduction to this volume (pp. 6-7), is the changing meaning of the word *individual* such that now it is the uniqueness, the distinctly different aspects of each person, that has come to be the most important characteristic of the individual. Previously these individual differences were usually seen by physicians as inconveniences that made the care of disease more difficult. In addition, patients themselves often tried to subjugate their personalities to the treatment plan, the hospital, or the doctor's schedule (as to many of the institutions of everyday life). Now they want their distinctness honored and served. They are more aware of their rights, and they use that language and speak frequently of their needs as individuals. Because physicians are also private individuals, these changes strike a responsive chord. Doctors are increasingly aware of the individual rights and needs of their patients, but do not yet have an established framework that allows these individual differences to become a legitimate aspect of their professional concerns.

A second reason that the subjective is surfacing now results from the recent changes in disease patterns. For acute diseases such as pneumococcal pneumonia, diagnosis and treatment depend very little on what things mean to the patient. Symptoms are so dire as to drive anyone for help, and, within limits, penicillin works, personal beliefs and values notwithstanding. But with chronic diseases like diabetes, arteriosclerosis, or hypertension, the situation is quite different. The presence and symptomatic expression of those diseases are determined, in part, by who a person is, by the personal meanings of things, by behavior. Diabetes may present itself differently depending on whether a patient is slothful or a long distance runner. Dietary habits influence the course of the illness, as does the patient's compliance with medical regimens. In other words, the nature of persons, how they act and interact with their environment, in addition to their genetic makeup, all exert an enormous influence on the presentation and course of the disease. In the treatment of hypertension, compliance is all: medication taken means blood pressure control; it is almost that simple. And patients do or do not take the medications because of beliefs about the efficacy or dangers of drugs, beliefs about stress, fears of stroke, and so on.

Discussions of these issues often emphasize psychosomatic illness. I have deliberately avoided that topic. The woman with metastatic carcinoma of the colon who did not follow up on her weight loss because it was pleasing to her may have profoundly affected her body. In the same manner, patients who do not take their medications— for reasons ranging from a desire to do things naturally to a general distrust of physicians—also cause things to happen in their bodies, sometimes with disastrous results. In these instances no esoteric relationship between psyche and soma need be sought. Indeed, recent studies in neuroendocrinology have begun to show evidence of the direct effect on body function of the personal meaning attached to events, objects, or relationships. On a simpler level, we are all aware of the chain of physiologic events set in motion in the body by the perception of danger. But what is danger to one is ecstasy to another. Only the meanings need differ.

The meanings we attach to things are, in large part, derived from our culture, the way the family was raised, relationships with family members, associations with other people, the roles we play, knowledge from other sources, day-to-day behaviors ("It's not me when I do not eat desserts"), past and present information from the body, and experiences of the lived past, including experience with illness and medical care. All these meanings add up to the needs, fears, desires, values, beliefs, and so on, that make up a person. This is not arcane knowledge buried deep in the inaccessible reaches of the human mind; in fact, most of it is there simply for the asking. But it is important to recognize that the information cannot be useful unless it is separated from the subjectivity of the physician.

THE PHYSICIAN
Art and Intuition
No measurement of the personal meanings of a particular patient can approximate the complexity of the meanings themselves. In this area, so-called objective tests or questionnaires are severely limited as tools for medical practice. Ultimately the physician must become

his or her own instrument. This is not an easy task, first because it involves using the physician's own knowledge, concerns, desires, fears, personal meanings (beliefs and values)—in short, the physician's subjectivity—to obtain information. And then it requires that the doctor separate out that information from himself or herself. Some physicians are highly skilled at extracting the history of their patients' illnesses from the matrix of personal meanings in which they are embedded. Those physicians can often predict the individual's behavior and obtain the cooperation of their patients in marvelous ways. Thus, we know it can be done. To dismiss such skills as intuition or art acquired at birth is simply wrong. In this context, intuition is frequently used the way "entelechy" was employed in the early days of embryology. Why did a limb bud appear where it did? It was entelechy, an informing principle. With hard work, better tools, and disciplined thought, the entelechy gave way to solid scientific facts. So it can be with intuition.

Art is another misused term. Unquestionably, some physicians are graced with talents that others lack, but once again, art is both improved by and is not a substitute for training. Charles Kossman, the cardiologist, was a master of the clinical arts. When I was a resident, I was startled to discover that despite his experience, he spent considerably more time listening to each patient's heart than I did. Perhaps that is why he usually heard more than I did. He would have pointed out that he was a careful listener and only perhaps an artist. Too often we try to write off certain talents as innate because we are not willing to put in the hard work required for their mastery.

Inner States

There are also the inner states—fear, for example—that occur in a doctor by virtue of taking care of patients. When a physician is called *subjective* it is generally in this sense that the word is applied, and most often with a pejorative connotation. Used in this fashion, it means that the doctor is "too involved" with patients and is unable to disengage his or her feelings from the clinical situation. Identification with patients that is too close causes us to have pain whenever something hurts them and to feel that we have lost a piece of ourselves when they die. Learning to become separate and not to identify too closely with patients is a necessary part of becoming a physician.

Those inner states—the feelings produced in the doctor by the patient's emotional responses to experience—have great diagnostic and therapeutic utility, but to use them well requires considerable learning, experience, and skill. We are forever urging our students to use their own feelings to understand their patients, but our request that they use their feelings is an unfair demand (born of our ignorance), and we ask it much too early in their careers. When young physicians become angry at a patient or are erotically aroused, they are not likely to ask, "Why is the patient trying to anger me or arouse me?" Usually those doctors simply become upset. Even asking someone what he or she feels usually brings a set of explanations for a feeling rather than a pure statement of feeling. The validity of feelings as information is undeniable. But considering how often medical students check and recheck an electrocardiogram, it is unlikely that they will learn early on to take action on the basis of an internal state known only to themselves, which hopefully reflects an internal state of the patient possibly not even known to the patient! It would be fairer if we first taught medical students simply to hear what patients say before we ask them to use their feelings.

Knowledge of Meaning

What is required to understand patients' personal meanings is the physician's acquired knowledge of the world of meanings. This includes not only what things mean to the doctor personally, but also what the doctor has learned about what things mean to others. Unfortunately, doctors, like other people, tend to act as though what is important to them personally and what they believe has the weight of objective knowledge. That failing can be overcome, and doctors can learn to hear the patients' personal meanings by learning appropriate skills.

Learning what things mean to patients is necessary for the most pragmatic reasons. The history of a patient's illness cannot be adequately assessed without separating the meanings the patient has assigned to the symptoms from the symptoms themselves. For example, it is difficult to get an accurate story of chest pain from a patient already convinced he has heart disease; and too often doctors are in the position of evaluating the patient's conclusions about an illness ("I'm always getting throat infections") instead of the illness itself (recurrent neck or throat pain). In the treatment of disease the influence of personal meanings is no less important. As I noted above, patients take medications or not, consent to surgery or not, rest or not, and so on, because of the meanings of things to them, not solely because of objective facts. (The same thing is true of physicians when they are ill.)

ATTENTIVE LISTENING

Most personal meanings (both the significance of events and their importance) are conveyed through the spoken language. Body language and other visual cues may be helpful, but the main message is conveyed by speech. Space does not permit more than a brief reference to the importance of a trained understanding of the patient's spoken message, but a few points can be made. The word choice of a patient tells the attentive listener how speakers picture themselves in relation to symptoms, other events, objects, or people. Verb choice can show the patients to be active or passive in the face of events—they can be "put in the hospital" or they can "go to the hospital." Adjectives and adverbs as well as tonal emphasis tell how the speaker values things. And valuative language is used about everything, so that the attentive listener learns the palette of values used by the patient—bright and sharp, subtle or subdued, and so on. Knowledge of word choice, generally characteristic of the speech of an individual, can then help in the evaluation of reports of pain or the description of other symptoms.

Conversation is virtually always logical, revealing a system of premises leading to conclusions. Premises may be spoken or unspoken, and they tell the listener what the speaker knows of the world and the structure of his or her beliefs. The patient who told his doctor, "I stopped taking the penicillin because I am allergic to dairy products," was not illogical; his premise was incorrect—"penicillin is made from dairy products, isn't it?" But that premise, part of the nexus of beliefs or implications that he perceives, determined whether he took a potent drug which determined whether his sinusitis subsided. Thus, meaning affected the outcome of an infectious illness by determining the patient's action. Even when the most important premises are unspoken, the logical flow of the conversation often suggests that a premise is missing. When a patient cannot be reassured and the conversation goes around in endless circles, it is frequently because an underlying premise is not being addressed.

Most listeners understand the speaker by knowing what they, the listeners, would mean if they used those words or spoke in that manner. That kind of untrained listening may be satisfactory for ordinary conversation, but it is inadequate for revealing the potential value of the spoken language in medical practice. There, the listener must learn to hear the patients' meanings in the words, usage, and manner of speaking. I have spent the last number of years studying the skills involved in attentive listening and how they can be taught. Most students are surprised at the amount of clinically useful information that can be conveyed even in short conversations. (It is something like looking through the microscope for the first time at an ordinary drop of pond water and being amazed at the complex life teeming beneath its everyday, taken-for-granted surface.) For all these reasons, I believe language and communication skills should be a fundamental part of the medical student's education.

When people are sick they are removed from their normal activities and spheres of influence, that is, disabled, in part by the effect of the disease on the body and in part by its meanings. In the 1950s, for example, patients with heart attacks might be disabled by persistent angina or congestive heart failure. Even in the absence of those complications such patients were also disabled by the need to stay in bed for six weeks (a belief of the times) and the understanding that after a heart attack one had to give up an active life and lead a sedentary existence—a meaning commonly attached to myocardial infarction in that era. See how different things are now. Patients may still suffer persistent angina or congestive heart failure, but they are almost never confined to bed for long periods. And many of them are more active and in better physical condition as a result of their myocardial infarction than they ever were before. Those changes came about not because of fundamental advances in therapy, but largely because of the changes in the meaning of the disease that were initiated when President Eisenhower showed that a person could be president after a heart attack. That experience would suggest that even when a disease cannot be cured, patients might be helped by changing the meaning the disease has for them.

Actually, this is done all the time, although usually without any awareness of the process. Consider the patient who comes to the doctor distraught because of the "melanoma" he or she has just found. The doctor says that it is a wart and cures the patient of a fatal illness by simply changing its meaning. You may think the only thing involved there were fears, but things are fearful only because of their meanings. Changes in meaning also involve physicians and their attitudes toward particular diseases, and patients who have such diseases. We are more optimistic about breast cancer, but attitudes have not changed that much for carcinoma of the lung; yet statistics do not bear out the differences. Such changes in the meanings of a disease are often not based on scientific evidence. The point is that if meanings that change without conscious effort can have such a profound effect on the well-being of patients, then personal and group beliefs and values could be changed as a determined therapeutic act. It does not matter that the intervention was directed at the person and not the disease; the person may be made better, and that is the point of it all. Thus, as knowledge of personal meanings has vital diagnostic value, it also has great potential therapeutic value. The area must be explored and understood, made into disciplined, teachable knowledge, and then taught.

We teach medical students to think scientifically and to use objective knowledge in the service of medical care. The presentation and course of human illness occurs through the interaction of biological systems of disease and patients' personal meanings and behaviors. What we teach students, by and large, covers only the first part of that equation. How can we correct that omission? Thinking about subjective information and making value decisions are different from reductive or analytic thought. The anecdote is often dismissed as a source of medical information because it is not scientific. But life is made up of anecdotes, and they have proven to be enormously useful in the education of our values and in teaching us to think about values. The Bible is a series of stories and the parables have a clear-cut mission; both succeed remarkably well in transmitting shared personal meanings in a culture. When we put anecdotes aside in medicine we pay a price. The anecdotal does not disappear from the doctor's life when his or her teachers disdain it; instead it simply disappears from professional view and is lost to systematic and disciplined use. Here, then, is another area for the investigator or teacher of medicine, and it will be rich in rewards, because it is both new to medical education and vitally necessary.

Most of what was presented here should be obvious. What has kept it from an honored place in medical science, education, and practice is its subjectivity. And that is the case because for science and objectivity to win the hard fought battle to enter medicine and move the spectacular distance forward that has occurred, the foil, the enemy that had to be conquered, was values and subjectivity. But that is really a red herring. This paper is really not about subjectivity, it is about personal meaning. The issue here is very simple. The time has come for personal meanings to gain their rightful place in medicine.

Clinical Medicine as a Science:
A Commentary on Eric Cassell

Ernan McMullin

Is clinical medicine a science, properly speaking? The question is hardly new. One can imagine it being debated in the ancient Greek medical centers when Aristotle's austere notion of science as an eternal and necessary knowledge of universals was first taking hold. In recent decades, as clinicians have turned more and more to laboratory tests on patients' bodily states, and as disease has come to be understood as a biochemical disorder or a biological infection, it has become tempting to suppose that the age-old question has found a simple answer. Clinical medicine becomes more reliable, more like a proper "science," as it takes on the shape of a theoretical, experimental discipline akin to biology or physics. And the training of the clinician, if this is correct, must approximate more and more closely that of the laboratory researcher.

It is this fairly widespread perception of the present status and future course of clinical medicine that Eric Cassell wishes to challenge. He does so by describing the "uses of the subjective" in medical practice and by arguing that these uses take one well beyond the laboratory stereotype of the biologist or physicist. I am inclined to agree with this general point, and I suspect that very few clinicians would in the end dispute it.[1] But I am uneasy with his choice of the term *subjective*.

It is not just that *subjective* has become almost a pejorative term, so that to speak of clinical practice as a subjective affair might seem to challenge the evident objectivity of its results. This objection could be met, in part at least, by distinguishing between different senses of the word *subjective*. More important, perhaps, is that Dr. Cassell's observations on the nature of clinical medicine do not neatly fit under the heading he has chosen. While they do concern the subjective in some of its many senses, the distance he wishes to place between clinical medicine and the classical model of theoretical-experimental science derives from much more than the uses of the subjective. The term *personal meanings* is also problematic: *personal* and *meaning* are at least as multifaceted as *subjective*, and the variety of points that Cassell makes does not lend itself to summary under a single title like this one.

These same points arise in other contexts. If one were to ask about the scientific status of sociology, history, psychology, engineering, or architecture, very similar issues would emerge.[2] None of these disciplines quite fits the neat paradigm of physics or biology, and there is an almost incurable tendency to think of physics and biology as the models to which other disciplines must be compared if they are to count as "science" proper.

THE SUBJECTIVE

I will begin with a few remarks about the term *subjective*. Since knowledge is by nature bipolar, involving both subject and object, there is a sense in which *all* knowledge is subjective, that is, it pertains to a knowing subject. It is likewise objective in the same broad sense, since it necessarily has an object even if that object should happen to be the product of imagination only. When philosophers speak of the "intentionality" of the knowledge-act, it is this peculiar duality that they are principally addressing. But this sense of *subjective* is too broad to be of service in making the sort of discrimination between different types of knowledge that Dr. Cassell has in mind.

In ordinary usage, the term *subjective* most often takes on the negative connotation, already alluded to, of a knowledge-claim which reflects the particularities of the knower rather than of the object.[3] It would, then, be an unreliable guide to the nature of the object. By contrast, an objective piece of knowledge is one which does what it purports to do, that is, it conveys in reliable fashion that aspect of the object about which a claim is being made. Provided that the aim of an utterance *is* to make a truth-claim, objectivity is obviously something desirable, and subjectivity, in this sense, is to be avoided. If one were to say of a particular clinical judgment that it is *subjective*, in this sense of the term, such a remark would ordinarily be critical in intent. It would suggest that the judgment reflects the bias of the clinician rather than the true state of the patient. Rather than introduce a suffix to indicate this particular way of drawing the objective/ subjective distinction, one might simply use the terms *reliable* and *unreliable*. Since the presumption is that clinical knowledge ought to be as reliable as possible, this sense of *subjective* obviously cannot help us in the analysis of good clinical judgment.

A third way of using the distinction is to discriminate between psychological states, to which only the knower has direct access, and physical states, which are in some sense public. To make this sort of distinction, one has to separate the psychological and the physical in a way which philosophers have endlessly debated since Descartes first made this a central issue. I shall avoid these questions here, important though they are to anyone who wishes to be exact in this use of the disputed term. When a patient says that an arm feels funny, or that he has had a particular dream, this is a subjective claim in the sense that it reports on his own subjectivity; it concerns events to which no one else has immediate access. Does this mean that they are beyond verification, unreliable, subjective in the second sense above? Not necessarily, though indirect modes of verification (Is this person usually truthful? Is he likely to show bias in this context?) have to suffice for people other than the subject himself. (The subject can, in favorable cases, have complete assurance about the reliability of his reports about his own psychological states; in some cases, however, as Freud among others has reminded us, he might have to distrust them.) One can be objective/reliable about one's own subjectivity, and one can take steps to be as objective/reliable as possible in regard to claims bearing on the subjectivity of others.

Is there something particularly subjective about interpreting the *language* of a patient in comparison to measuring the iron levels in his blood? Dr. Cassell's essay on the uses of the subjective stresses the importance to the clinician of a "trained understanding of the patient's spoken message" (p. 164). Yet it is not easy to say why the interpretation of language (the "hermeneutic act," as philosophers like to call it) should be called subjective, if the recognition of a pneumococcus on a microscope slide would not be. It cannot be because a psychological state is being reported: "I jog regularly" needs interpretation just as much as "I feel a throbbing sensation in my back." Nor is the subjectivity of the clinician engaged in an essentially different way; a special knowledge-skill is required, but then that would also be true of the bacteriologist identifying the pneumococcus.

But as Cassell points out, the interpreter is in a sense trying to sort through the subjectivity of the speaker. That is, he can attain to the object, to the matter reported, only as this is refracted through the subjectivity, the mind of the speaker. The subjective here is a sort of screen that imposes its own structures on what comes through, and the skill of the interpreter resides in discerning what lies beyond it. This would not, however, entitle one to speak of the skill as a subjective one, nor of the interpretive act itself as subjective; although subjectivity is uniquely involved in the act of interpreting the language of another, the involvement is not such as to warrant introducing yet another sense of the term *subjective*. Perhaps a different rubric should be used for treating the special problems associated with the interpretation of language.

In the remainder of my comment I propose to separate out three problems to which Dr. Cassell is directing our attention under the capacious canopies of *subjectivity* and *personal meaning*. Each can be situated within classical discussions of the scope and nature of science. And each problem corresponds to difficulties that arise if one tries to force clinical medicine into the framework classically attributed to a natural science.

INTERPRETING THE LANGUAGE OF ANOTHER

The historian has to rely on written documents as his starting point; the social scientist must frequently turn to spoken testimony for his evidence. Thus, the interpretation of the language of others, of people often remote in culture or in time, is central to the work of historiography and social science. It is this, above all, which led so many in the past century to argue that there is a sharp distinction between the natural and social sciences, or, to put this in another way, that the model of science applicable to physics is inapplicable to, for example, sociology.

I shall not take sides on this issue here. But there can be no doubt that the skill of interpreting the language of another is of a very different sort from the skill of recording or interpreting a chemical experiment. The clinician, like the historian, is trying to make an objective assessment of a situation by listening carefully to what another has to say of it. Instead of working directly on the organism, as a biologist might, he is attempting to gain the information he needs by looking, as it were, through the eyes of someone else who can give this information. Sometimes the information-content is easy to extract ("The accident happened at noon today"; "I had measles when I was seven years old"); at other times, considerable effort may be required in order to determine what exactly is being conveyed ("The pain was really terrible"; "I just don't feel like eating").

The information is of many sorts. The most important has to do with the patient's history: specifics of illness, nutrition, lifestyle, and the like. Another has to do with the patient's character. This sort of information is harder to get; it is usually not sought directly, but may be tentatively constructed over a period of time on the basis of conversational hints and responses, known habits, and so forth. Knowledge of character is especially important in the prescribing of therapy, but can also be relevant in the diagnosis of certain sorts of ailments.[4] Information about the patient's values (one part of Cassell's "personal meanings") comes somewhere between; it, too, would seem to be more relevant to the therapy stage, not only because knowledge of the likely responses of the patient is often crucial to prescribing a regimen, but also because what counts for the patient as health or an acceptable quality of life or unacceptable pain can be all-important to the clinician in deciding what treatment is to be proposed. Its relevance to diagnosis is less obvious, but is no less real.[5]

In interpreting the information given, associations (perceived implications as well as emotional overtones) can be important. For an individual who has experienced its effects on someone close to him, chemotherapy may have quite different associations (not only emotive, but also in terms of correctly perceived consequences) than it would for someone to whom it is only a hopeful remedy. Once again, this seems more relevant to prognosis and treatment than to diagnosis.[6]

The language of the clinical history is inevitably less precise than that of the laboratory report, and Dr. Cassell is warning against the temptation to underrate the clinical history in consequence.[7] And he also advocates more attention to ways of taking histories in the training of the clinician-to-be. For he believes that the knack of hitting on the right question, of picking up nuances of meaning, of uncovering relevant aspects of the patient's personality, can be taught, or, at the very least, that their importance in clinical work can be emphasized more than it currently is, so that aspiring clinicians will take these skills seriously and work to acquire them.

A SCIENCE OF PARTICULARS?

Aristotle insisted that science was of the universal, that it deals with universals, not particulars. The "new science" of Galileo left aside the "impediments" of the natural order and idealized to universal laws and theories to which the particular was expected to correspond to a progressively greater extent. Thus, although the experimentalist deals with particular instances of planetary motion or gas compression, he attempts to formulate laws which hold for planetary motion or gaseous pressure-volume ratios in general.

In this perspective, what is one to make of engineering or architecture? There one has to adapt to the particular; one must build a road across a particular terrain or fit a house into a particular urban location. These are by convention called applied sciences, because they take over the abstract universals of the physicist and apply them to specific situations where the "impediment" can no longer be idealized away. But is this skill of dealing directly with the particular a part of science proper? Or should it be called an "art"? And what is one to make of the historian's labors? Most historians would balk at calling their work "applied science," the relevant sciences here presumably being psychology, sociology, and the like. Though they may on occasion venture to make generalizations, their primary duty is to the singular, to the illumination of the particular event or the individual character.

The resonance with medicine is evident. The physician's concern is with the individual patient. He will make use of whatever the sciences of biochemistry, physiology, and the like have to offer him. And in his own role as researcher, it is to these sciences he will mainly contribute. But to a clinician, the universals of the researcher are a means to an end, that is, the healing of a particular person. Like the engineer, he must make the best use possible of the most up-to-date general knowledge that bears on his problem; but his success will be estimated not by the empirical laws he discovers or the theories he formulates, but by his success in hitting on the right means of helping *this* person.

Dr. Cassell's emphasis on this point (which has been made before[8]) stems from his concern that the growing involvement of the physician in research may lead him to misunderstand his primary vocation, which is not to the sick in general, but to particular sick people. And he may, in consequence, neglect or underestimate the skills that are needed for dealing with the individual sick person. These are different skills, just as those of the engineer are different from those of the physicist, and those of the historian differ from those of the sociologist. The issue here is not one of developing a good rapport with the patient in order to further effective therapy; nor is it a question of making the patient feel that he counts as an individual in his own right rather than just as another liver or heart. The issue is primarily a cognitive one: what means must the clinician adopt in order to understand (diagnose) the state of *this* organism and, if necessary, restore it to health?

The particularity of the patient's value system, to which Dr. Cassell points, is only one part of a much wider issue. One patient is a jogger; another has parents who died of a heart disease; another may have been exposed to radioactive material in his work at a weapons plant. These are not primarily matters of value assessment. But they may be crucial to the medical problem the clinician faces. And they may not neatly fit into any of the universals he possesses. Their conjunction may, indeed, create a situation entirely novel as far as he is concerned. The ability to deal with this situation and the hedging of judgment that it entails are characteristic of the good clinician.

Dr. Cassell advocates the "systematic study" of the sorts of particularity to which the clinician will be exposed. If his recommendations are heeded, physicians will be taught a disciplined and systematic approach to their patients' subjectivity as a basic part of medical education. This emphasis on systems in the approach to the particular is somewhat troubling. It is as though Dr. Cassell is still, despite his emphasis on the irreducible particularity of the clinical case, trying to impose system and order of a kind that can be taught. Is this too much of a concession to the classical ideal of scientific respectability? It sounds as though universals are being readmitted through the back door.

Part of the problem may be that he is mingling two issues that I have tried to keep apart: the interpretation of the subjective report and the particularity of the clinical situation. The former of these can be approached systematically; one can, as Dr. Cassell notes, help the student learn how to "read" a patient's testimony, what to look out for, what to discount. The problem here is not with particularity, but with penetrating the language of another. It is true this language may be particular in some ways, that the associations for this patient of this word may be quite special. But there is no systematic way of approaching particularity of this sort. This is, in part, what makes it particular. The engineer, the historian, the clinician have to learn to live with the unexpectedness of the particular. It is not to be circumvented by some new "skill of the particular."

For all skills must rely on analogy with cases previously encountered. It is the perception of likeness between some aspect of the problem situation and a situation already handled that serves as the clue. And we do not yet know whether it is possible to systematize this perception by means of explicit rules. This brings us to the third difficulty in conforming clinical medicine to the classical stereotype of science.

THE COMMUNICATION OF TACIT SKILLS

In the classical accounts of science, it seemed as though scientific method could be set down in a series of explicit rules of a formal sort, a logic of demonstration or confirmation. But the project of reconstructing such a logic met with little success. Polanyi, in particular, showed that many of the skills of classification and assessment that the scientist needs are tacit ones, incapable of being set out in formal, explicit rules. It would thus be widely accepted among philosophers of science today that the identifications made by bacteriologists or radiologists, for example, involve a skill of tacit knowing that must be taught by dint of repeated practice rather than by a manual. Similarly, the formulation of hypotheses, the weighing of alternative theories, and many other aspects of the scientist's work, require cognitive skills that are learnt obliquely, by watching how others proceed and trying at first to imitate and then to surpass.

Clinical medicine is thus not peculiar or any less scientific merely because its skills are often of this sort. It may seem as though research medicine is comfortably intersubjective and methodic, or that its skills can be communicated in a neutral and direct way. Were this the case, the contrast between it and clinical practice would be sharp indeed. But the skills requisite for medical research include a large tacit component, and thus the separation between the two, though real, is not as great in this respect as might at first sight be supposed.

Nevertheless, clinical medicine is, to an unusual degree, intuitive, in the sense of involving skills that are difficult to specify in terms of explicit criteria. The history of recent attempts to construct computer simulations of clinical judgment is instructive in this regard. The internist program at the University of Pittsburgh is particularly interesting because it attempts to simulate as closely as possible the judgments of a particular clinician, Dr. John Myers. To "simulate" means two things here: to make the same judgments on the same data as Myers would, and to follow the same criteria and relative weightings that he does, to the extent that these can be made explicit. But the project has shown that these criteria are extraordinarily difficult to make explicit; one certainly cannot argue to them in any direct way. Satisfactory simulation, in any save limited areas, seems to be a long way off.

If these skills of assessment are hard to specify and therefore to teach in the conventional "blackboard" way, the difficulty is very much greater when one comes to the conduct of clinical dialogue. Attempts have been made to formulate questionnaires with branching lines of questions so the interview could be structured in a formal way. This could be helpful up to a point. But in more complex cases, as Dr. Cassell reminds us, a sensitivity to nuances of language and to shading of personality is indispensable. This is very hard to teach, and it is often regarded as an inborn gift.[9] The ability to discern meaning and character is assuredly much more developed in some than in others and is allied with personality pattern, but Dr. Cassell is right to emphasize that one can learn to be more effective in this discernment.

One learns this, however, not from explicit instruction as much as from perceptive involvement with good clinical work. One also listens, as Dr. Cassell puts it, to parable and anecdote. But in the end, as he admits, those doctors who have successfully learned how to cope with the subjectivity of the patient's testimony did not learn to do this in medical school but from their ultimate teachers, sick persons. Could they have done so in medical school? How far-reaching a change would be required in the methods of medical education?

Although Dr. Cassell's essay leaves us with questions about the precise role that personal meanings play in accurate diagnosis, and about how to inculcate the skill of reading these meanings, it does give us something of an enlarged understanding of what is meant by "science." To propose medicine instead of mechanics as the paradigm of science would be too radical; the origins of the concept "science" are too firmly associated with notions of demonstration, causal understanding, and maximally secure knowledge to make this move a plausible one. But clinical medicine does provide a useful challenge for the theorist of science, accustomed as he is to the simpler fare of physics. For in clinical medicine, many of the most interesting issues of contemporary theory of science flow together: the status of the hermeneutic disciplines, the means to a reliable knowledge of the particular, the communication and assessment of the tacit skills so important in all forms of knowing. The mix of problems Cassell describes will certainly draw increasing attention from philosophers.

Notes

1. This point has been made by a number of recent writers, most notably by Reiser (1978a).

2. For a discussion of subjectivity and the social sciences, see Diesing (1972).

3. There are some complications here in the context of those theories of knowledge (those of Kant and neo-Marxism, in particular) where knowledge either inevitably or appropriately reflects the cognitive structures of the knower. I am taking the simplest variant here and assuming that to reflect the particularities of this knower is not to convey the nature of the object, but in fact to distort it. But this would need a more detailed treatment than I can offer here.

4. Cassell describes diabetes, arteriosclerosis, and hypertension as diseases whose "presence and symptomatic expression ... are determined, in part, by who a person is, by the personal meanings of things, by behavior. Diabetes may present itself differently depending on whether a patient is slothful or a long-distance runner.... In the treatment of hypertension, compliance is all ... " (pp. 160-161). Slothfulness is a matter of character; long-distance running is a matter of habit. It might be simpler to treat them under these headings rather than as personal meanings or values.

5. Of course, psychoanalysts claim that most illness has an emotional component in which values and associations may play as important a causal role as do bacteria and viruses in infectious diseases.

6. In Cassell's example of the two patients suffering from pneumonia (p. 155), the fact that one lost both parents to the disease and sees it as fatal, whereas the other patient sees it as easily treatable, would, so far as I can see, affect diagnosis only in that the former would be more likely to construe his own illness as pneumonia and might thus exaggerate the expected symptoms.

7. See Reiser (1978b).

8. This point is forcefully made by Gorovitz and MacIntyre (1976).

9. Cassell objects to writing off clinical skill as art or intuition. But to describe it in terms of art and intuition is not necessarily to see it as innate: art requires training; intuition often needs patient apprenticeship. Clinical

skill is indeed an art; once again, devotion to the classical objectivist notions of science must not lead us to draw overly sharp boundary lines between art and science. See McWhinney (1978).

Bibliography

Diesing, P. 1972. "Subjectivity and Objectivity in the Social Sciences." *Philosophy of the Social Sciences* 2: 147-65.

Cassell, E.J. 1985. "Uses of the Subjective in Medical Practice," pp. 151-166 in this volume.

Gorovitz, S. and MacIntyre, A. 1976. "Toward a Theory of Medical Fallibility." *Journal of Medicine and Philosophy* 1: 51-71.

McWhinney, I.R. 1978. "Medical Knowledge and the Rise of Technology." *Journal of Medicine and Philosophy* 3: 293-304.

Reiser, S. 1978a. *Medicine and the Reign of Technology.* New York: Cambridge University Press.

_____. 1978b. "The Decline of the Clinical Dialogue." *Journal of Medicine and Philosophy* 3: 305-13.

Part III:
Directions for Philosophy
in Medicine

Humanistic Education and
the Physician's Art

Max Black

THE PROJECT

The question I propose for discussion is: How might the humanities help to improve medical training and medical practice?

I start with a confession of ignorance concerning much that is relevant to this tangled theme. This violates the conventional introduction of a speaker by reference to his titles and special qualifications. But if my qualifications for talking about medicine are slender, I console myself by hoping that better-informed readers may correct my deficiencies and help me to improve the tentative proposals that follow.

One difficulty with my initial question is that its chief terms, *medicine* and *the humanities,* are vexingly problematic. Medicine and the humanities are what philosophers sometimes call essentially contested concepts,[1] that is to say, honorific and hence contentious appellations. Medicine is agreed to be a Good Thing; and the enticing label of "the humanities" could hardly fail to stand for something worth having: all of us would like to be humanists and to have the services of superbly qualified doctors. Yet humanistic specialists cannot confidently say what a good humanist is, and at the Conference on Changing Values in Medicine there was much disagreement concerning the definition of a good doctor. So my question looks like a quixotic effort to connect two shifty variables.

I shall try to alleviate the embarrassments of this disconcerting situation by formulating explicitly my own initial assumptions, so that the reader may check both my premises and the conclusions I draw from them. I shall say something about the physician's art, then rather more about the contributions that the humanities might make to the training of physicians. I shall end with a few modest but relatively specific curricular proposals. All of this can be no more than a preliminary sketch for later elaboration.

Let us start then with the assumptions.

OUR PRESENT CONDITION

I hope the members of this first group of assumptions will seem obvious or even banal. The first assumption is that we are in a period of possibly unprecedented changes in economic, political, and social structures. A decade ago, Alfred Kazin said, "This is ... the most revolutionary era in recorded history, the most thoroughgoing transformation of established habits of living and thinking that has ever been known" (1967). Five years ago, the *New York Times* published an alarming piece entitled "Old Planet, New World," by F.M. Esfandiary (identified as a teacher of long-range planning at the New School for Social Research and the author of *Telespheres*). "The entire world," he says, "is at the beginning of a historic turning point. We are moving up to the post-industrial age" (1979). Ahead of us is an age of "telecommunication," "tele-education," "tele-medicine," "telefarming," and so on. That versatile prefix *tele-* salutes a dystopia in which nearly everything will be "telefacted"[2] (my own neologism), an age of universal action at a distance.

One may hope that Professor Esfandiary's peep into the future is an implausible and somewhat hysterical fantasy. But is it altogether implausible? Anybody born before the First World War has seen the fantastic become the commonplace. One need not be a septuagenarian to remember trams pulled by horses, or to recall the thrill of first scratching the "crystal" of a primitive radio set with a "cat's whisker." (We managed in those days without radar, sound movies, zippers, jet planes, lasers, the Pill, and the other paraphernalia of present affluent existence.) It is surely reasonable to expect further technological innovations that will make our present discussion as quaintly old-fashioned as the Farmer's Almanac.

I agree with Professor Esfandiary that we may expect extensive applications of computer technology to medical practice.[3] That may well be a Good Thing. Why spend as much time as medical students now must in laboriously memorizing inert facts if computers can do that job faster and more reliably? Even that famous "intuition" of the experienced diagnostician may eventually yield to computerized "simulation." Up to a point—an important qualification—projected three-dimensional pictures of the patient's condition, together with a resumé of his relevant medical history, may eventually elicit from a well-programmed computer a better basis for diagnosis than a practitioner's hunches.

My second assumption is that the massive changes in prospect are largely unpredictable. John Maynard Keynes once said of the impending Second World War: "The First War produced Hitler. What can we expect after the Second? Hyenas?"[4] Could he or anybody else have predicted the Holocaust or Hiroshima? And after another world war, what can we expect? The survival of cockroaches perhaps? We are and will remain irremediably ignorant about apocalyptic future events; the only reliable lesson to be drawn from the past is that the future will be in some ways unexpected and horrible.

Let us also remember (with what *Punch* once memorably called "a glimpse of the obvious") that the present age, partly owing to its accelerating instability, is marked by radical and pervasive disagreement about many basic factual and normative issues. The Conference on Changing Values in Medicine has provided a good illustration of controversy about even as relatively straightforward a question as whether students can be taught to become good doctors. (Here and throughout I use *teaching* in the sense of "helping to learn.") I should have thought it indisputable that we can significantly help students to become good doctors, whenever we agree about our goals and are willing to take enough trouble. We know that sufficiently talented beginners can be helped to acquire such sophisticated skills as those needed for piano playing, playing chess, reading Sanskrit, or controlling airports. Then why so much controversy about the feasibility of medical education?

A contributory cause may be that our own education has conditioned us to view skepticism as a hallmark of sophistication. We live in what Disraeli a century ago called an age of "craving credulity." Intellectuals and professionals are volubly opinionated: we believe the incredible and disbelieve the obvious.

In his *Decline and Fall of the Roman Empire*, Gibbon wrote: "The various modes of worship, which prevailed in the Roman world, were all considered by the people as equally true; by the philosopher, as equally false; and by the magistrate, as equally useful" (1957, Chap. 2). That fits our present condition, at least in the nondictatorial states. Any teacher knows the blank looks that greet a reference to the Bible, or the disbelief aroused by a suggestion that there are objective moral principles. We encounter in our students and colleagues cynicism rooted in ignorance, oddly coupled with uncritical acceptance of dogma. Students think of themselves as hard-bitten skeptics, but what they believe often beggars belief: witchcraft, telekinesis, TM, anything but what has been established beyond reasonable doubt by centuries of sustained effort.

If this is an accurate diagnosis of our present condition, a serious question arises as to how far we can help beginners to cope with so much anticipated instability and uncertainty. Well, the least we can do is to discard academic baggage that will probably be useless.

(A useful maxim might be: Teach only what human beings can do better than computers.) We might well try harder than we now do to produce versatile rather than well-stuffed graduates, those who can still learn after fifteen years of cramming. If there are teachable skills of learning and problem-solving, we should do our best to communicate them. If we can graduate highly adaptable and resourceful people who can cope rationally with high unpredictability and uncertainty, we shall probably have done our best for them. But if we continue to mimic Jehovah by trying to produce others in our own images, we shall, in certain important respects, be miseducating the next generation.

THE PHYSICIAN'S ART

Much of what I would like to discuss under this heading has already been adequately covered by other contributors to this volume, so I can be rather brief.

I want to support the other contributors who have described the doctor as being primarily the practitioner of an art, in the Greek sense of *technē*, and so as being a craftsman rather than a scientist. A doctor is not and cannot be a scientist, not even an applied scientist; this is too pretentious a designation for a professional who is basically a consumer of the findings of medical research. A physician's distinctive vocation is to be a master of the complex of practical skills that identify him as an expert craftsman or artist.

The skills in question are social ones, depending essentially upon cooperation by the patient. The physician's art is not a solitary affair like plumbing or painting. Being a doctor is like being a chess player: one needs a partner. Without the patient's cooperation, medical expertise and skill are useless. When a patient refuses to do what his doctor thinks advisable, we have a medical hitch or a failure.

It follows that the healing art is largely a communicative or persuasive art of inducing the patient's remedical actions. It should therefore be viewed as a rhetorical art, in the older, nonpejorative sense of rhetoric as the art of persuasion. A doctor is more like a teacher or an advertiser than like an engineer: the patient, unless he is a child, a lunatic, or is temporarily unfit to provide informed consent, must be helped to understand what needs to be done in order to help himself. Of course, I do not wish to say that medical practice involves only communicative and rhetorical art: a doctor has more to do than talk and persuade.

As a rhetorical art, medical expertise demands judgment and skill grounded in experience. But above all, it depends on imaginative sympathy, no less than upon reliable scientific knowledge. This is one reason, I believe, why no computer can be a good doctor. For a computer cannot conceivably respond with resourceful and sympathetic understanding to human problems.

Consider the case of the doctor portrayed in John Berger and Jean Mohr's splendid book, *A Fortunate Man: The Story of a Country Doctor* (1967). As we follow this remarkable country doctor in his daily work, we are insistently reminded of how much more than scientific know-how is needed for somebody working as a professional in and for a community. Berger says that his subject "is acknowledged as a good doctor." When some of the patients were asked why they though so well of him, "they would say that he was straight, not afraid of work, easy to talk to, not standoffish, kind, understanding, a good listener, always willing to come when needed, very thorough." It is interesting that nothing seems to have been said about his medical qualifications, which were presumably taken for granted. In that particular English village, the doctor's contributions to the health and happiness of his community depended at least as much upon his human qualities as upon his technical expertise.

Let us agree now, if we can, that the medical art is also inescapably moral. Paul Goodman once said, with pardonable exaggeration, that engineering is a branch of moral philosophy. The epigram applies equally well to medical practice. I am not thinking here of the dramatic moral issues of abortion, euthanasia, and the like, which, for all I know, may now be adequately handled in the new courses offered in some forward-looking medical schools.[5] I think rather of the moral aspects of everyday interaction between doctor and patient. Considerations of truth and humbug, honesty and deception, respect and coercion, continually arise. I have known doctors who handled such matters tactfully and gracefully, without worrying about the difficult theoretical issues posed by such topics as informed consent, the patient's right to relevant information, the merits and demerits of detailed knowledge of risks and uncertainties, and the like. But I hope the reader will not share the fashionable anti-intellectual view that rational discussion of such issues has little to contribute to the relevant practical skills of rational persuasion. Here, as elsewhere, misologists, despisers of theory, can be self-serving manipulators of their patients.

IMPLICATIONS FOR MEDICAL TRAINING

My first assumption under this heading is that the college preparation of prospective physicians should be available and useful to all students, regardless of their future careers.

In his article on Reason in the great French encyclopedia of 1779, Diderot said, rather boldly, "[N]ous sommes hommes avant d'être chrétiens"—we are human before we are Christians. Perhaps we should insist, in the spirit of this remark, that students are human before they are medical students. It might indeed be a good thing to discard the concept of "premedical" education altogether.[6] Then we might bend our best efforts to encouraging the emergence of educated and decent human beings without neglecting the special needs of those who may end up as doctors.

Such a shift of emphasis is desirable, because it is so hard to tell in advance which students will eventually become doctors. Of the fraction of prospective doctors who manage to enter medical school,[7] a good many will become researchers or medical administrators or will turn to another occupation. Conversely, some very able physicians have entered the medical profession late in life. We should not base a substantial segment of college education on the needs of a special and largely unidentifiable minority. We can, however, reaffirm that we deserve doctors who are at least well educated. It is a serious question whether current premedical training on the whole serves that purpose or rather tends to divert students from it. I think the latter.

I propose that one explicit aim of the preparatory curriculum should be the development of general intellectual skills; for instance, the skills exercised by numerate persons who have mastered basic mathematical concepts and understand the powers and limitations of measurement and statistics, but are not necessarily good calculators. The goal should be to produce knowledgeable amateurs who know how to improve, refine, and develop what they have learned. I think in this connection of the graduates of the great French technical schools, the *hautes écoles normales*, who can in short order learn to run a bank or a government department, on the job, without much preliminary specialized training. (It might also be worth studying the records of such academics as the Oxford philosophers who performed so well in the British intelligence services.)

I propose also that a substantial segment of the basic curriculum should concern the development of powers of expression and interpretation. The literacy envisaged should extend far beyond what is commonly taught under the rubric of "English composition" (and only occasionally required for admission to medical school). All of us sorely need better training in skills of reading, writing, speaking, and understanding: too many professionals—not only doctors—fail to meet respectable standards of comprehensive literacy.

In line with my previous insistence upon the moral dimensions of the physician's art, I also propose some provisions for serious ethical study. There is no dearth of relevant materials: the contention that there is nothing to learn from over two thousand years of ethical controversy is too silly to be worth discussing.

HUMANISTIC EDUCATION

Let us now consider how the humanities might help in such a program for producing literate, morally responsible, and versatile professionals. We had better start by agreeing, if we can, about the meaning we want to attach to the problematic and controversial label of *humanities*. Nowadays, an unabridged dictionary is apt to treat *humanities* as a mere umbrella term for literature, history, philosophy, and sometimes also the "fine arts"—that is to say, for disciplines or departments that cannot be plausibly classified as either science or mathematics. A college campus will be apt to have some ramshackle building serving what Americans call "the humanities." (The English prefer to speak of "arts," in opposition to "sciences," while the French prefer the label of "les sciences humaines.") Such a building is often regarded as a tolerated enclave for "the finer things of life," not to be taken seriously by tough-minded devotees of intellectual study. Thus, a young engineer may be advised to take a little "culture," rather than yet another course in machine-drawing, because it won't hurt him to relax while listening to a harmless old fogy burbling about Homer.

If the humanities are still regarded as somewhat esoteric indulgences, teachers of the humanities are themselves partly to blame.

Consider the following remarks by R.B. Hutchins:

> The crucial error is that of holding that nothing is more important than anything else, nothing central and nothing peripheral, nothing primary and nothing secondary, nothing basic and nothing superficial. The course of study goes to pieces because there is nothing to hold it together. ... We have nothing to offer as a sound curriculum except talk of personality, "character," and great teachers, the slogans of educational futilitarianism.
>
> (from a talk at Yale in 1940, quoted approvingly in I.A. Richards 1955)

Many of our best humanists will concede that teaching for nonprofessionals too often remains an exercise in "futilitarianism."

Yet the rich and diverse history of humanism includes ambitious and coherent educational programs that are not futilitarian in Hutchins's sense. The term *humanitas* itself, coined by Cicero as a translation of the Greek *paideia*, has a noble pedigree. In the second century A.D., the grammarian Aulus Gellius said:

> Those who have spoken Latin and have used the language correctly do not give the word *humanitas* the meaning which it is commonly thought to have, namely, what the Greeks called *philanthropia*, signifying a kind of friendly spirit and good-feeling towards all men without distinction; but they gave to *humanitas* about the force of the Greek *paideia*, that is, what we call *eruditionem institutionemque in bonas artes*, or "education and training in the good arts." Those who earnestly desire and seek after those are most highly humanized (*maximi*

188 / Max Black

humanissimi). For the pursuit of that kind of knowledge, and the training given by it, have been granted to man alone of all animals, and for that reason it is termed *humanitas*, or "humanity."

(quoted from R.S. Crane 1967, vol. 1, p. 23)

Here an ambitious and coherent educational program is postulated. Renaissance educators believed that human beings are born as mere animals, needing for the full development as men "the arts of humanity," that is, "those branches of learning [*disciplinae*] by means of which we separate ourselves from the way of life and the customs of animals and are restored to humanity" (Quintilian, quoted in Crane 1967, vol. 1, p. 31).

The humanists of the Italian Renaissance in the fourteenth to sixteenth centuries never doubted that there is a distinctive human essence, a sheaf of potentialities that need cultivation by means of special arts or disciplines. The supreme educational goal, one might say, was to transform *Homo sapiens* into *Homo humanus*, to convert mere beasts into urbane, civilized, and morally responsible human beings. This inspiring program stamps the Renaissance as one of the great formative educational movements of Western civilization. (It would be interesting, if we had time, to see how the educational ideals of the Renaissance were adapted and modified in the later humanistic programs that led to the establishment of the German gymnasia and the somewhat different adaptations of Renaissance ideals that animated the reform of public school curricula in nineteenth-century England.)

Yet, for all its appeal, the Renaissance conception of humanistic education now needs to be modified, if only because it rested on philosophical assumptions that are now unacceptable. We need to discard the assumption, shared by all Renaissance humanists and by most of their admirers and imitators since, that there is such a thing as a so-called human essence, that is to say, a set of necessary and sufficient properties that distinctively qualify its bearers as human. Almost as implausible is the view, as old as Aristotle, that identifies the alleged human essence with rationality. Erasmus said, "What is the proper nature of man? Surely it is to live the life of reason, for reason is the peculiar prerogative of man" (quoted in Abrams 1971). In somewhat the same spirit, Locke said "[Reason] stands for a faculty in man, that faculty whereby man is supposed to be distinguished from beasts, and whereby it is evident he much surpasses them" (1929, iv, xvii, 386). And Charles Darwin, who did so much to discredit the apparent radical discontinuities between men and beasts, could still say, "Of all the faculties of the human kind, it will be admitted, I presume, that Reason stands at the summit" (1871, 1, ii, 46). It will be noticed that neither Locke nor Darwin go as far as Erasmus and countless other thinkers in urging that Reason or rationality is the

sole prerogative of humankind, but hold only the weaker position that humans surpass all other animals in rationality. History might persuade us that even this weaker position is exaggerated: human irrationality is too endemic for complacent self-congratulation.

There are, I believe, good reasons to reject the historically influential commitment of humanists to the existence of a human essence. There are no qualities, as far as I can see, which individually or together are the sole prerogative of human beings. What makes us human is rather a syndrome of features, among them, to be sure, the possession of a distinctive kind of body, consciousness, power to reason and make rational choices, but also the capacity to feel, to pretend, to imagine, to express intentions, attitudes, and valuations, and to articulate all these varied aspects of human life in shared languages.

No simpler view will do justice to the observable complexity of normal human beings. It is well enough to make so much fuss about that remarkable chimpanzee Washoe who, if its trainers can be trusted, has reached the intellectual level of a somewhat retarded five-year-old.[8] A monkey will count as humanly developed only when it can do such things as invent jokes, gossip, praise and blame actions from a moral standpoint, and much else. If Washoe or any other animal ever exhibits such a syndrome of capacities, we shall then have to admit that persons need not have human bodies. The same goes for computers: if they can eventually be programmed to justify their actions, reproach their makers, and so on, the nature of their "hardware" will be unimportant. We shall then have to accept them as artificial human beings.

If this conception of the human syndrome is on the right lines, any humanistic program of education that is committed to the development of a supposedly unique human essence will need drastic amendment.

HUMANITIES AS YIELDING DISTINCTIVE KNOWLEDGE

A principled effort to revitalize the teaching of the humanities in order to restore them to their deservedly central positions in education will need to come to grips with the debilitating dogma that refuses the title of genuine knowledge to anything but the fruits of "scientific method." An adherent of such diluted positivism or "scientism" is likely to view humanistic studies, to the degree that they do not aspire to be scientific, as no better than genteel adornments to the serious cognitive business of life. But scientism is no longer a respectable position, if it ever was.

Humanistic study and any educational program using its products are necessarily committed to methods of understanding and interpretation that cannot be called scientific in any plausible sense of that label. Whether you agree with this quite unoriginal contention will, of course, depend upon the concept of scientific method with which you operate. Some philosophers of science, who conceive of all scientific disciplines as aiming at the condition of physics, insist that a perfected science can be no respecter of persons, places, or times. Such a science should aim, like physics, at finding universal principles, indifferently applicable to all instances of highly general categories such as "matter," "motion," "electrical charge," and the like. But even respectable physical disciplines, such as geology, oceanography, or meteorology, are committed to a distinctive interest in particulars of special human concern (*this* earth, *these* oceans). A defensible methodology of science must accept this: there is nothing pejoratively "impure" about the desire to have detailed knowledge of topics as absorbingly interesting as neurophysiology. Interest in a particular configuration of matter—for example, my own body and its uniquely instantiated properties—for the sake of reliable information and accurate prediction, even if unlikely to yield general conclusions, is not on that account to be denigrated as unscientific.

Yet a scientific interest which is in this way "idiographic" and not "nomothetic" (Rickert's labels for sciences respectively emphasizing particular facts and universal laws) still fails to come to grips with questions that concern each human being profoundly. The universe that I experience is not the impartial space-time continuum of contemporary physics, perceived in a kind of God's-eye view that treats all places and times as indifferently worthy of notice. For me, the particular place now occupied by my body has a preeminent interest as the seat of felt pain and pleasure and the origin to which direct perception is referred. Similar remarks apply to the time I recognize as "now," and to the experienced feeling of duration (Bergson's *durée*). The space-time in which each of us lives and moves has knots and grain; that is one reason why we need such token-reflexive words as *now, here, there,* and especially *I, you,* and *we.*

Yet science has no use for the distinction between me and you. The point can be illustrated by the following joke. A man complains to his friend about his accumulated misfortunes: he has broken his leg, his son is in jail, his wife has left him, he has cancer, and so on, in a crescendo of woe. Each item's recital elicits the same response: "It could have been worse." When the sufferer bursts out at last with, "What could be worse than that?" the answer is, "It could have happened to me."

Had I the time, I would now make a similar point about a person's specific beliefs, attitudes, sentiments, and emotions at any particular moment, and would talk about the limitations upon their expression by general formulas. They are not to be thought of as incommunicable or ineffable, hidden within some private realm; on the contrary, we typically express or reveal our feelings and intentions, by words and involuntary gestures or symptoms. Now much of the educational value of the humanities consists precisely in the training they provide in the recognition, comprehension, and critical evaluation of such expressive behavior. The outcomes deserve to be called knowledge and insight, though unrecognized as such by some tough-minded scientists.

I shall resist a philosopher's temptation to talk at this point about the logic of singularity or the peculiar structure of a person's experienced world (his *Lebenswelt*). Let me illustrate the point more simply in the following way. Ivan Il'ich's death, in Tolstoi's wonderful story, concerned that man in a way that is not captured by talk about the death of Il'ich, somebody identified from the outside by a proper name or a definite description. It sounds atrociously callous to use here the joke formula: "It could be worse, it might have happened to me." But the idea so expressed is not silly, however hard it may be to formulate sensibly. The poignancy of individual existence and individual destiny is something each of us understands and feels: if we do not talk about it, that may be because there is nothing to be done about it. But it has been eloquently delineated in literature, history, and philosophy. One does not capture the nature of Shakespeare as a unique person by reciting facts about his being the son of a businessman or his having left his wife his second-best bed. In order to begin to know Shakespeare himself, one needs at least to read his works with imagination and love, or better still, *per impossibile*, to have been his fellow actor and friend. In such ways one may sometimes gain the kind of insight about human beings that can be shown but not stated. No amount of verbal description of a person, no photographs or CIA files or anything of that sort, can fully reveal what he is really like or can replace the insight yielded by direct encounter in friendship or hatred.

I would like to suggest that for anybody to be bereft of the aids to such knowledge of self and others as the humanities can provide is to be sadly crippled. While reading a philosophical paper at Oxford, G.E. Moore once used some blackboard formulas. H.A. Prichard, a formidable philosophical opponent, opened the subsequent discussion by saying, with a sneer: "Well, Moore, I never did understand all those Xs and Ys." To which Moore replied: "Really, Prichard? How disgraceful!" Perhaps this is the right tactic to shame students who are perversely proud of cultural deprivation. "Never heard of Jane Austen? Really? How disgraceful!" Or, less dismissively: "Really? What a shame!"

SOME CURRICULAR PROPOSALS

I pass on now to a few proposals, modest but perhaps useful, for curricular innovation. Since the science requirements for admission to medical school can be satisfied in four semesters, there is ample room in the undergraduate curriculum for some general education. I propose assigning part of this time to three units of course attendance. The first would be a year-long course that might be called "Methods of Inquiry," or perhaps, more explicitly, "Investigation, Evidence, and Proof." I think of it as a general intellectual service for all sophomores and juniors.

Such a course would discuss methods of discovery and procedures of intellectual justification, with special attention to how they vary from one discipline to another. There should be some elementary logic in it, and much discussion, analysis, and evaluation of informal arguments, expressed in ordinary English. Ample materials can be found in newspapers, advertising, political speeches, and textbooks. I would want to include some inductive logic and probability theory as well as an elementary introduction to statistical methods. Also a unit which might be called the "Ethics of Belief" (starting perhaps with William Kingdom Clifford's essay having that title, and also using William James's famous essay, "The Will to Believe"). It might be useful to include some material on the role of observation and experiment in the formulation and confirmation of scientific theories. I would emphatically wish to include a good deal of discussion of patterns of discovery and justification in humanistic studies—literary criticism, history, and philosophy.

This kind of course would be interdisciplinary, using materials from a variety of specialties—logic, philosophy of science, methodology, epistemology, and the many subjects labeled "philosophy of X." I think academics might enjoy developing such a course. If it went well, it might be highly beneficial to all undergraduates, whether or not they eventually landed in medicine.

A second-year course, which might be called "Meaning and Communication," would draw inspiration from the strong emphasis in Renaissance education upon language and speech. The materials would be largely taken from linguistics, philosophy of language (with special attention to speech-act theory), and rhetoric. Ethological studies of so-called animal communication would be relevant, as would illustrative materials from radio, television, and advertising. Emphasis would be upon varieties of expression and the distinctive powers and limitations of different media. There should be ample provision for practical exercise as well as sustained theoretical discussion.

Next, I would like to see every student urged to take a rigorous year-long course in what might be called "practical ethics." It might be designed as an exposure to the elements of moral philosophy, using a case study approach for raising problems that seriously agitate the young and their elders. Discussion of specific ethical predicaments could demonstrate the practical bearings of the competing moral systems of utilitarianism, emotivism, and the rest.

Finally, I should like to see all undergraduates without exception soak themselves for at least one year in some particular branch of the humanities, whether history, literature, or philosophy.

Since such a program would require altogether about one year's work, it should present no insuperable scheduling problems, even for preprofessionals.

Would this kind of program be apt to produce better doctors? Well, speaking as a past, present, and future patient, I would like my own physicians to be, above all, well trained and well informed enough to provide me with the kind of diagnosis and treatment that they would wish for themselves. But I would also like them to be exemplary human beings.

The kind of humanistic education for which I have been pleading might indeed help.

Notes

1. See W.B. Gallie's (1964) influential essay, "Essentially Contested Concepts."

2. Esfandiary's upbeat conclusion is "With intelligent planning and vision, we can now accelerate the evolution from obsolete industrialism to the marvels of a new age of limitless growth, abundance, leisure and indefinite lifespans."

3. For an example, see the brief report, "New Diagnostic Technique," in the *New York Times* (October 2, 1979), on "a new automated medical diagnostic technique for detecting pancreas, liver and intestinal malfunctions." With the new system, "analyses that previously required eight hours and the constant attention of a specially trained technician can now be done in one hour by an unattended machine."

4. I have been unable to find a reference for this quip, which I quote from memory.

5. Of the several textbooks now available, see, for instance, Beauchamp and Childress (1979).

6. Compare Lewis Thomas's (1978) attack on the present system.

7. According to Arnold Relman (1978), about half of the American students applying to American medical schools are admitted.

8. See, for instance, Linden (1976).

Bibliography

Abrams, M.H. 1971. *A Glossary of Literary Terms.* New York: Holt, Rinehart and Winston.

Beauchamp, T.L. and Childress, J.F. 1979. *Principles of Biomedical Ethics.* Oxford: Oxford University Press.

Berger, J. and Mohr, J. 1967. *A Fortunate Man: The Story of a Country Doctor.* New York: Holt, Rinehart and Winston.

Crane, R.S. 1967. *The Idea of the Humanities.* Chicago: University of Chicago Press.

Darwin, C. 1871. *The Descent of Man.* New York: D. Appleton.

Esfandiary, F.M. 1979. "Old Planet, New World," *New York Times,* October 12, p. A31.

Gallie, W.B. 1964. "Essentially Contested Concepts." In *Philosophy and the Historical Understanding.* New York: Schocken Books.

Gibbon, E. 1957. *The Decline and Fall of the Roman Empire.* New York: E.P. Dutton and Co.

Kazin, A. 1967. "Literature as a Necessity of Life." *New York Times Book Review,* July 30.

Linden, E. 1976. *Apes, Men and Language.* New York: Penguin Books.

Locke, J. 1979. *Essay.* New York: Clarendon Press.

Relman, A. 1978. "Americans Studying Medicine Abroad: The Distressing Facts." *New England Journal of Medicine* 299:887-89.

Richards, I.A. 1955. *Speculative Instruments.* New York: Harcourt, Brace and World.

Thomas, L. 1978. "The Pre-Med Syndrome." *Chronicle of Higher Education* 17, no. 14:48.

Environmental versus Biological Causation in Medicine: A Commentary on Max Black

Stanley J. Reiser

There is a uniformity of view about the scope and purposes of medical education today, despite Professor Black's apt characterization of our time as one of turbulence and change. This view has roots reaching back to the sixteenth century. It is based on a concept of people as machines and is wedded to a method of fact-finding which uses the experiment to uncover the causes of illness.

A notion that disease has a locus in the body, and that illness might be understood by demonstrating the relation between functional change and structural alteration in the body's fabric, was the principal legacy of the new anatomical school of learning that developed in the sixteenth century. Its origins were greatly influenced by the work of the Flemish physician, Andreas Vesalius, through his book, *The Fabric of the Human Body* (1543). The book transformed the medical understanding of normal human anatomy through its insistence that (1) anatomists, rather than their assistants, perform dissections; (2) statements of fact and hypotheses be tested not by reference to learned authorities, but by reference to nature; and (3) textual material be accompanied by accurately drawn illustrations. It also stimulated the study of the effects of disease on structure, which reached an influential plateau in 1761, when G.B. Morgagni completed *The Seats and Causes of Diseases Investigated by Anatomy*. This work, as its title suggests, asked physicians to conceive of diseases as having "seats" in the body, and to explain symptoms by tracing them to specific anatomical transformations that could be seen by the eye or felt by the hand. It convincingly argued that the best path to scientific discovery and clinical excellence was continual reference of lesion to symptom. It thereby introduced as a fundamental tenet of medicine the clinico-pathological correlation. Physicians applied this intensively during the late eighteenth century and into the nineteenth century in the pursuit of medical knowledge, using the scalpel as the main weapon of conquest.

The technology, but not the ideology, changed in 1855 when Rudolf Virchow's treatise, *Cellular Pathology*, appeared. It brought together a large amount of data, some already existing, others produced by Virchow, to demonstrate that the cell was the fundamental unit of biological life within whose borders the activities that maintained normal function and caused pathological change took place. As Virchow himself insisted, the question central to the study of pathology that had been posed to medicine by Morgagni—"Where is the disease?"—remained vital, and indeed was reinforced and emphasized by his work. Virchow transferred the site of study from organ to cell and substituted the microscope for the scalpel as the principal tool of the pathologist.

Today, such technology has taken us deeper into biological structure, but the key pathological question posed by Morgagni and Virchow continues to be asked by modern clinicians. For us, disease continues to have a "place" in the body.

This structural view of disease was also encouraged by the intensive exploration, beginning in the sixteenth century, of a powerful technique of testing facts in science—the experimental method. Like the anatomical method, this one entailed learning how things worked by analyzing matter into its components. Facts were generated and tested through experiments, which could be reproduced by the skeptical. Wherever possible, investigators sought to express the evidence gained from the experimental test in quantitative and graphic terms, which seemed to free evidence from human bias. The new experimental investigations of human nature sought to banish from scientific attention all considerations based on value, perfection, or meaning because these notions seemed out of place with the spirit of experimental inquiry, which sought to remain value free. As the twentieth century began, Karl Pearson urged the scientist to "above all things strive for self elimination in his judgments, to provide an argument which is as true for each individual mind as for his own" (1900, p. 6).

Those in medicine who have adopted these ideologies interpret disease basically as structural disruption and tend to exclude from medical learning and practice a view of illness as an intensely personal event whose aspects cannot be understood or dealt with solely by methods based on experimentation or measurements. The power of the subjective view of things, of the ability for imaginative participation or empathic understanding into the actions and works of others, is not the stuff on which the biologically oriented physician dwells. Accordingly, in the modern medical environment it is difficult to introduce disciplines such as the humanities, which explore the values, motives, and traditions that mold the purposes, duties, and warrants of medical care.

An alternative view of illness, one that reaches from the Hippocratic work, *Airs, Waters, Places,* to British physician Thomas McKeon's recent book, *The Role of Medicine,* asks why disease has occurred rather than how it operates once it is in place. Advocates of this position argue that health depends primarily on the control of environmental influences, including those that individuals fashion for themselves, rather than on medical interventions or knowledge of physiochemical mechanisms of body action. They believe the best approach to combating disease rests not so much on exquisite technical interventions into biological mechanism, but on efforts to learn how we are influenced by the environments we create. Inherent in this view is an attention to values, meanings, and aims—concerns that a concept of medicine as a technological intervention in a biological machine tends to exclude.

Professor Black sees the art of communication as an essential dimension of the medical art and would exert considerable efforts to enhance the physician's skill in this sphere. I am in agreement. A good clinician is a good teacher. I also find congenial his suggestions to introduce courses in evidence and medical ethics into the undergraduate curriculum. But he neglects medical education. The humanities, like communication skills, cannot remain the captive of college classrooms: they must also be taught at medical schools and brought into the medical clinic as well.

Professor Black makes an interesting comment in reference to the medical art: "The skills in question are social ones, depending essentially upon cooperation by the patient.... Without the patient's cooperation, medical expertise and skill are useless" (1985, p. 184). He thus implies that a change of life can lead the patient to better health, and that the skills in communication and persuasion which he accords such high value are to be marshaled to induce such health-giving changes. He appears, then, to be comfortably at home with the environmental view of health and medicine.

But there is an ambiguity in this important statement of Professor Black's which can lead to significantly diverse interpretations of the appropriate role of the doctor's intervention into the personal life of a patient. Does it mean that doctors should guide the patient to a good life—as doctors see it? Or that doctors should help patients realize their own goals, even if doctors think them inappropriate? Or that doctors should refuse to treat uncooperative patients? How does one draw the line between cooperation and submission? As we learn increasingly more about the aspects of environment and lifestyle which influence illness, we shall be under ever greater pressure to exercise authority over the right of patients to live as they please. How far should intervention into the preferences and habits of individuals be carried by health care practitioners? To what extent should they become involved in the formulation of public policies to limit disease-generating behavior?

The environmental view, with its prescription to alter social structures and habits of living, raises questions that are clearly within the boundaries of problems traditionally dealt with in the humanities. In contrast, in a view of medicine that equates disease and structural change, that relies for evidence on the experimental method, the humanities appear to have a lesser role. In this latter ethos, technical answers seem the key answers.

Those who teach the humanities in medical school must continually show why technological answers in medicine are often incomplete and why methods of fact-finding—in addition to those of the biological sciences—are needed to decide many of the questions raised by illness. In addition, they must also caution advocates of an environmental approach to illness about the dilemmas of implementing this view. Whether the humanities can successfully meet such tests in medicine will determine their value to those who seek to help the sick and preserve the well-being of the healthy.

Bibliography

Black, M. 1985. "Humanistic Education and the Physician's Art," pp. 181-195 in this volume.

Morgagni, G.B. 1960. *The Seats and Causes of Diseases Investigated by Anatomy*. New York: Hafner.

Pearson, K. 1900. *The Grammar of Science*. London: Adam and Charles Black.

Vesalius, A. 1543. *The Fabric of the Human Body*.

Virchow, R. 1855. *Cellular Pathology*. Berlin.

Philosophy and Medicine

John Ladd

INTRODUCTION

The purpose of this essay is to explore in a rather general way the relationship between philosophy and medicine: what it has been, what it is, and what it ought to be. Anything I can say here about this complicated subject will be impressionistic and programmatic. It will also, of course, be controversial, for like every philosophical subject the question of the relationship of philosophy to medicine is itself controversial. I hope, therefore, that my comments will be taken in the spirit intended, that is, that they will be regarded as speculative and suggestive rather than as definitive or final.

At the outset, it must be freely acknowledged that apart from heroic attempts to link philosophy and medicine by appealing to the fact that Aristotle's father was a physician or that John Locke was a country doctor, historically the relationship between these two disciplines has in fact been more of a nonrelationship. That is not to say that it has been unfriendly; it has simply been a relationship of mutual "benign neglect": benign, not in the medical sense meaning harmless, but in the ordinary, nonmedical sense meaning kindly, gracious, and mild. Philosophers and physicians have treated each other like friendly neighbors who, having nothing in common, pass each other on the street with a friendly nod of greeting and then go about their business happily ignoring each other.

There are well-known reasons for this historical nonrelationship between the two subjects. Philosophy, since the time of the ancient Greeks, has been oriented more toward mathematics and physics, as far as the sciences are concerned, than it has towards medicine or even biology.[1] Medicine, on the other hand, has had closer ties with religion than it has had with philosophy.[2] The association of medicine with religion has a long history and continues even today; a cynic might attribute their relationship to a common fondness for "miracle, mystery, and authority," conceptions that are generally anathema to philosophers.

In our day and age, however, there may be more affinities between philosophy and medicine than there are either between philosophy and the physical sciences or between medicine and religion.[3] Indeed, recent developments in both fields suggest that a rapprochement between the two disciplines is long overdue. In philosophy, we find a rapidly growing interest in the philosophy of the biomedical sciences, as well as the development of new methodologies and analytical techniques in the areas of what might be called "practical philosophy" (i.e., in value theory and ethics). These and other recent changes in philosophy auger well for more serious philosophical involvement in the problems of medicine. Similarly, the development of medicine as a rational discipline, that is, as a science, may be expected to result in its being weaned away from religion and becoming more like other sciences that are the objects of philosophical inquiry. It hardly needs to be pointed out that the many spectacular changes in medicine during the past few years—both from a theoretical point of view, as a science, and from the point of view of its practical and social importance— have created a spate of new problems and issues that cry for clarification through philosophical analysis. The new medicine presents many exciting challenges for philosophy and, as a philosopher, I hope that philosophy will be able to contribute to a deeper understanding of the puzzling theoretical and practical problems confronting contemporary medicine.

For purposes of the present inquiry, I shall treat philosophy and medicine as intellectual disciplines rather than as institutions or ways of life. When considered as an intellectual discipline, the most obvious thing about medicine is that it is grounded in science or, indeed, it is itself a science, and that medical practice bases its authority on the claims of medicine to be a science. Its scientific character is clearly what marks off medicine from other kinds of health care projects such as those undertaken by laymen at home and in the community, or by mystics, faith healers, and magicians. One of the aims of this essay is to show how the notion of medicine as a science generates a variety of theoretical and practical problems that should concern both philosophers and physicians. For once medicine is accepted as a science, philosophers will naturally begin asking such questions as: What kind of a science is it? Is there a special logic or methodology peculiar to medical science? How does medical science relate to medical practice? How does medicine, considered as a science, relate to the health and well-being of individuals and of society? Although these questions may appear to be easy to answer, I shall try to show that the answers are really very complicated and also that they are interconnected. For example, the answer to the first questions about medicine as a science will have a logical bearing on the sorts of answers that will be given to the other questions about medical practice, about the responsibilities of the physician, and about the role of medicine in social decision making. I hope that the kind of logical investigation I shall outline here will convince skeptics of the critical importance of a philosophy of medicine for an understanding of both the theoretical and moral aspects of the dilemmas that are the inevitable by-product of the successes of modern medicine.

WHAT PHILOSOPHY IS AND WHAT IT IS NOT

Before turning to more substantial matters, I need to explain briefly my conception of what philosophy is and what it is not. For if it is made clear at the outset that there are certain things that philosophers are especially equipped to do and others that they are not at all equipped to do, then the reader will not entertain false expectations. To begin, philosophers should not be expected to be priests, lay preachers, or lay prophets. There is no philosophical handbook with ready-made prescriptions for all the complicated moral dilemmas of modern medicine. To expect a philosopher to be prepared to solve all of a doctor's moral problems is to confuse philosophers with casuists or ethicists, the modern equivalent of a casuist. Unlike the latter, a real philosopher does not set himself up as an expert or authority on moral questions after the fashion of a tax lawyer who tells a client in detail what he can or cannot do. Instead, the philosopher's role is to be a searcher after truth, that is, to be an investigator, a questioner, and a prober. For that reason, a philosophical approach to medicine may be expected to be theoretical, speculative, and skeptical, rather than dogmatic, authoritative, and determinative.

What, then, is philosophy in the sense intended here? To answer this question, I shall refer to Wittgenstein, who writes in the *Tractatus*: "Philosophy is not a body of doctrine but an activity. Philosophy does not result in 'philosophical propositions,' but rather in the clarification of propositions. Philosophy aims at the logical clarification of thoughts" (1961, 4:112).[4]

Another philosopher, Immanuel Kant, subscribes to almost an identical notion of philosophy: "Philosophy cannot be learned, for a philosophy that is conclusive and universally valid does not exist. One can only learn to philosophize" (Cassirer 1912, band II, S.320).

From the conception of philosophy as an activity, it follows that, generally speaking, it is a second-order discipline, a reflective inquiry aimed at clarifying various other modes of thought. As such, it has no subject matter of its own; it consists, instead, of critical reflections on other subjects, that is, of philosophizing about other subjects. Thus, perhaps with a few reservations, philosophy may always be thought of as a philosophy *of* something, for example, philosophy of science, philosophy of law, philosophy of language, philosophy of history, or philosophy of art. In the same vein, the principal aim of philosophy of medicine is to philosophize about medicine, that is, medical science and medical practice.

It may help to be more specific about what is meant by *philosophizing*. The purpose of philosophy is understanding: it seeks to understand ideas, thoughts, conceptual schemes, modes of reasoning, and the like, by clarifying them and showing their interrelations. The kind of clarification sought through philosophizing is generally known as conceptual analysis.[5] Insofar as philosophizing aims at the clarification and explication of concepts, it is applied not only to individual concepts, but also to the logical relationships between concepts and to the conceptual framework in which sets of concepts are cast. As I shall presently explain, this kind of philosophical analysis inevitably and necessarily implies a critical evaluation of the concepts to be analyzed and the conceptual structures in which they are framed.

Historically, and by its very nature, philosophy is problem oriented.[6] The distinguished philosopher C.I. Lewis used to tell his students that philosophy is simply the residue of unsolved problems. He held that when problems are solved they drop out of philosophy and are incorporated into one of the sciences, so that all that is left in philosophy are the problems that have not yet been solved. It is not necessary to agree with all of this, but Lewis was certainly right to emphasize the problematic character of philosophy. One should expect to get problems and questions from a philosopher rather than answers. For much the same reason, philosophy is inexorably controversial: it is born in, thrives on, and ends with controversy.

So that there will be no misunderstanding of the view taken here of the nature and function of philosophy and, in particular, of philosophy as it applies to medicine, a few further comments about the critical evaluation of concepts are in order. Philosophers tend to take two different kinds of positions with regard to the relationship of philosophy to its subject matter, that is, the ideas and concepts to be analyzed.[7] One view, which may be called the passive conception of philosophy, is that philosophy takes its subject matter as fixed and given, that is, as providing pre-established data for analysis and for use in testing the adequacy of the philosophical theory that is offered to explain them.[8] Accordingly, a proposed analysis is not permitted to affect or change the data in any way—at the risk of rendering the analysis in question circular. Among philosophers of this persuasion, the preferred method for refuting a proposed analysis is to find a counterexample that will prove the nonequivalency of the analysans and the analysandum.[9]

The other position, which I consider more fertile and productive, may be called the active conception of philosophy. According to this conception, any sort of philosophical analysis of a concept, in the sense of clarification or explication, is bound to change it. For this reason, the so-called data for philosophical analysis are never "pure" or "hard," but are always molded in one way or another through the analytical process itself. One could say that there is a sort of a feedback effect between analysis and its subject matter.[10] If philosophical analysis is active rather than passive, as I believe it should be, then philosophizing can have a practical impact on how we think about a subject; critical analysis and evaluation show when and how concepts need to be restructured, when they may be dispensed with, and when new ones have to be created. Thus, an active conception of philosophy implies that philosophers should not only seek to interpret the world but should also try to change it.[11] Still, as I have pointed out, the method of philosophy is indirect rather than direct, for it operates critically only through the analysis of concepts or, broadly speaking, through the critical articulation of thoughts and thinking processes.

QUESTIONS FOR THE PHILOSOPHY OF MEDICINE

Having briefly discussed what philosophy is and what its relationship to medicine should be, we are in a position to review briefly the kinds of questions that are appropriate for the philosophy of medicine. In addition to those mentioned earlier, a philosopher of medicine may be expected to address such questions as the following: What is the purpose and nature of medicine? What kind of concepts are the concepts of disease, health, treatment, and cure? What kind of science is medical science? How do values enter into medicine? And what is the relationship between medical science, medical practice, and ethics?

If, by investigating questions like these, philosophy can lead to a better understanding of the conceptual apparatus of medicine, then it should help us not only to cope with some of the urgent dilemmas facing modern medicine, but also to resolve more general issues regarding, for example, the autonomy of medicine, its status as a technology, the authority of the doctor, and the place of medical science in medical decision making. In the course of this essay, I shall make a few suggestions about some of these issues, but I will focus primarily on one particular issue: the conceptual relationship between medicine as a theory and medicine as a practice. The theme to be developed is that it is logically impossible to keep the theoretical and practical aspects of medicine separate; therefore, one of the principal tasks for the philosophy of medicine is to clarify and explicate the relationship between these two sides of medicine.[12]

THE LOGIC OF MEDICINE: THREE MODELS

The easiest way to bring out the conceptual and logical problems relating to theory and practice in medicine is to examine three models of medicine which represent three different ways of viewing the nature and function of medicine. These models correspond roughly to different historical stages of the development of medicine as a rational discipline. My formulations of them are imaginative reconstructions and make no pretense to historical accuracy or philosophical profundity. My main object is to show the various directions that a philosophy of medicine might take and, indeed, has taken at various times. I shall call these three models (1) the *technē* model, which I associate with Aristotle; (2) the applied science model, which I associate with John Stuart Mill and logical positivism; and (3) the practical science model, which I shall contend is a more accurate model for contemporary medical theory and practice than the other two and which I believe will be a more appropriate model for the development of medicine in the future.

The Greek philosophers and most of their pre-Renaissance successors did not find in medicine the same kinds of philosophical puzzles that they encountered in mathematics and physics or even in politics and theology. It is easy to see why Greek philosophers found mathematics and physics so engrossing, for these subjects give rise to many tantalizing philosophical puzzles, puzzles relating, for example, to the ontological status of numbers and to the relationship between geometry and physics. Politics and government present interesting puzzles about power, authority, and the social order, while theology provides philosophically interesting puzzles concerning the nature of possible relationships between an infinite, omnipotent being and the finite world of his creation. But medicine, as the Greeks knew it, did not present the same kinds of intriguing philosophical puzzles that were encountered in these other areas. Medicine was simply identified as a craft, a skill or *technē*, and its problems were thought to be practical rather than theoretical. Accordingly, it was placed in the same category as architecture, shipbuilding, and the military art. We must begin, therefore, by examining more closely what the Greeks meant when they called medicine a *technē*.

Medicine as Technē: The Aristotelian Model

Although both Plato and Aristotle have theories about the nature of *technē*, Aristotle's discussion in the *Nicomachean Ethics* is the best source for our purposes.[13] Aristotle defines *technē* as intellectual excellence connected with doing and making. In introducing his discussion of the intellectual virtues (or excellences), he begins by dividing ratiocination, rational thinking, into two categories, which he calls scientific (*epistemonikon*) and calculative (*logistikon*).[14] Scientific thinking is concerned with invariable and universal principles, whereas calculative thinking is concerned with particular and variable things where generalizations hold only "for the most part." Scientific ratiocination is held to be certain and demonstrative, while calculative rationcination is held to be inexact and experimental.

According to his analysis, *technē*, in contrast to science, has three distinctive attributes. First, *technē* uses calculative rather than scientific ratiocination. Second, the outcome of *technē* is an action (a doing or a making) rather than a belief. Third, *technē* has an end. Aristotle says that the end of medicine is health and that the role of the physician is to use his *technē*, his expertise, to promote and to restore health. In doing so, he deals with individual cases or particulars, rather than with general principles or universals. Thus, *technē* is experimental rather than theoretical. In all these regards, medicine can be compared to strategy, the *technē* of generals, or economics, the *technē* of the household.[15] For any of these skills, the quality of the result provides the standard by which the quality of the activity and the degree of skill is judged. Although those who possess the *technē* have specialized expertise, a layman is capable of evaluating the expertise simply because he knows the value of the result. Just as the layman is able to know from the results who is a good shipbuilder or a good general, so he is able to tell who is a good doctor and to determine whether or not the doctor has the requisite *technē*.[16]

The undervaluation of the theoretical or scientific side of medicine probably reflects the state of medicine of the time. The development of modern science in the sixteenth and seventeenth centuries, especially in anatomy, physiology, and chemistry, made Aristotle's first assumption about medicine invalid, for it became increasingly evident that medicine has a scientific base.

Medicine as Applied Science: The J.S. Mill Model

With the recognition of the scientific side of medicine, it is obvious that another model is needed. I shall call this new model the applied science model.[17] A good description of this model is to be found in John Stuart Mill's *System of Logic* (1872) under the heading "The Logic of Practice or Art." Although Mill did not explicitly apply his model of the logic of practice to medicine, it is easy to do so and, in fact, his model corresponds very closely to a certain conception of medicine that still prevails and has many adherents.

Mill presents his conception of the logic of practice or art in the form of a syllogism consisting of three parts: the major premise, which is an end supplied by art; the minor premise, which is supplied by science; and the conclusion, which is an imperative or rule of some kind.

In his exposition of this practical syllogism, Mill writes:

> The art proposes an end to be attained, defines the end, and hands it over to the science ... Science then lends to Art the proposition (obtained by a series of inductions and deductions) that the performance of certain actions will attain the end. From these premisses Art concludes that the performance of these actions is desirable and finding it also practicable, converts the theorem into a rule or precept (1872, book vi, chap. xi, para. 2).

It is easy to see how this model can be applied to medicine. The end may be identified as health (the elimination of disease, etc.). The intermediate minor premises are provided by medical science, and the conclusion consists of imperatives and maxims of medical practice, that is, procedures and treatments. This interpretation conceives of medicine as an applied science—that is, as medical technology—and as such, it has a logical structure analogous to that of engineering. Let us examine this model more closely.

The first thing to observe is that in Mill's account the distinction between science and art is absolute and qualitative; it is not a matter of degrees. The underlying assumption appears to be that science itself is, in modern terms, neutral and descriptive; it is connected with behavior only through the adoption of an end, represented in the assertion that the attainment of a given end is desirable. Mill's contrast between the assertion of ends and the establishment of scientific facts makes it easy to move a step further and conclude that the selection of ends is always subjective and relative; instead of being determined by reason or science, the choice of ends is determined by personal preference, by the marketplace, or by an authority (medical, institutional, or political). Mill himself, a good utilitarian, did not go that far. But the built-in subjectivity of the applied science model, the technology model, lends plausibility to the view that medicine, as a technology, receives its ends from the outside and therefore should be adapted to whatever ends the doctor, the patient, or society elects to adopt. Accordingly, in a market economy, medical technology becomes a commodity that is used to meet the demands of consumers, whatever they may be. This view of medicine provides a theoretical foundation for medical consumerism. In addition, when medicine is conceived of as an applied science or technology, it loses its claim to autonomy. To paraphrase a famous utterance of Hume, it becomes a slave to the passions of others, that is, to their preferences and desires.[18]

The particular kind of separation of science and value that is epitomized in Mill's account is not due simply to a misguided view of values, but also to an overly narrow conception of science itself, a conception that construes science as value-neutral and value-free. This last point and its implications for philosophy of medicine will become clearer when we examine the final stage in the philosophical separation of practical science from science proper, namely as it emerges in the philosophy of science developed by modern logical positivism or "logical empiricism." Logical positivism typically espouses three principles, any of which, in my opinion, makes a coherent account of medicine as a practical science quite impossible. These three principles are:

1. The covering law model of explanation: the theory that in order to give a scientific explanation of an event it must be subsumed under a covering law (Hempel 1968, chap. 5; Hull 1974, pp. 87-100).
2. The rejection of the notion of a "logic of discovery": the process of discovery must be kept separate and distinct from the logic of justification.
3. The doctrine that science is value-free and value-neutral: considerations concerning Is and Ought, or Fact and Value, must be kept separate and distinct so that science will be entirely objective and empirical.

All three of these principles have recently been under attack from various quarters. I want to emphasize that even if we grant that they hold for physics, none of them is compatible with any kind of working idea of medicine, with the notion of medicine as a practical science. In any case, we must give serious consideration to the thesis that no adequate theory of medicine is possible unless these three principles are rejected or, at least, are qualified in important respects.[19]

Another Model: Medicine as a Practical Science

Bearing in mind their application to medicine, I shall now describe some of the elements of the model of a practical science, which I contrast both with the *technē* model and with the applied science (or technological) model. The points at issue in this contrast will emerge clearly if we compare the modern idea of medicine with the notion of applied science already described. To begin with, medicine does not simply tell us how to procure health or absence of disease; it also tells us what health is and what disease is. As a layman, I take for granted that it is good to have a healthy heart, but only a medical person can tell me what a healthy heart is.

In medicine, as in other practical sciences, ends and means are inextricably interwoven. Terms like *health* and *disease*, as well as more particular medical concepts, have both a value and a descriptive component: on the one hand, health is something desirable and disease

is something undesirable, while, on the other hand, the determination
of how these concepts are to be applied requires specialized medical
knowledge. On closer inspection, it should become clear that, contrary
to the positivist doctrine, many of the basic concepts of medicine have
both a value and a scientific dimension. Concepts such as function,
equilibrium, homeostasis, abnormality, deficiency, and immunity, and
disease words ending in *itis* or *osis* all are value-laden concepts; that
is, they involve reference, either directly or indirectly, to conceptions
of what ought to be rather than simply of what is, was, or will be.[20]
Indeed, the very notion of a medical problem is value-laden, itself,
as is the correlative notion of a solution, for the determination that
there is a problem and what it is, as well as what an acceptable solution
to it would be, necessarily involves an evaluation of some sort.[21] On
closer inspection, we will soon see that the precise articulation of
the value dimension of different medical concepts is a complicated
matter, for there are many ways in which values enter into medicine.

Let us now turn to the second positivist thesis, the thesis that there
is no such thing as a logic of discovery. On the face of it, this thesis
does not appear to fit medicine very well: in medicine the ratiocination
required for the solution of a medical problem (e.g., a clinical
diagnosis) must be systematic in the sense of following certain lines
and procedures—this amounts to a logic of discovery. A good diagnostician, for example, uses algorithms as described by Alvin Feinstein (1973, 1974) and other methods elaborated in the recent work
of Schaffner and others.[22]

Finally, the covering law theory of explanation does not appear
to provide a satisfactory amount of the kind of explanation that is
required in medicine. One facet of this theory is the symmetry principle,
that is, the assimilation of the logic of explanation to the logic of
prediction. Medical diagnosis is better conceived as a form of
explanation rather than as a form of prediction, for a diagnosis may
be thought of as satisfactory if it simply identifies a certain necessary
condition of a disease, for example, the presence of a bacillus or tumor.
For this purpose, it is unnecessary to establish the sufficient conditions
of the disease as would be required for a prediction.[23] Furthermore,
in medical diagnosis we are interested in finding an explanation of
a particular fact (a sign or symptom) about a particular person in
a particular situation, and it may not be possible to find exactly the
right covering law to use in explaining this kind of fact in all its
specificity. Sometimes particular facts can be better explained by
relating them to other known facts about the person in question than
by appealing to a general law. That is why a clinical history is so
important in diagnosis. In addition, even general facts about a certain
disorder or derangement are often explained by other general facts,

(e.g., about a certain kind of obstruction), without reference to a covering law under which they could be subsumed. We know, for example, that a certain chemical deficiency leads to hypertension, even though we cannot specify the mechanisms that connect them causally (Gorovitz and MacIntyre 1976).

In view of the objections to the older models of medicine, and simply from the point of view of philosophy of science, we need to develop a new model. In addition to meeting the objections already mentioned, the new model should help to explain how an intellectual discipline like medicine can have the properties of both a science and an art (or *technē*). That is, it should be able to show in detail how the scientific and the value aspects of medicine are interconnected logically, and to set out the logical consequences of their interconnection. The development of a new model along these lines is a challenging task for philosophy of medicine.

MEDICINE AND MEDICAL ETHICS

These suggestions concerning the philosophy of medicine also have important implications for medical ethics, for the thrust of my argument is that value questions and scientific questions cannot be sharply separated in medicine as the *technē* or the applied science models require. Some further discussion of the interrelationships between medical, value, and ethical questions will help to bring out the radical nature of the program that I propose.

We may begin with medical concepts: The physician is a medical scientist and pursues his practical clinical activities by reference to concepts of medical science. These include the general concepts of disease, explanation, diagnosis, and treatment, as well as more specific concepts. As I have indicated, the concepts themselves, in terms of which the physician's problems and solutions are couched, have a value dimension. In addition: the connections between medical science and practice, and between medical science and value (or ethics), are not casual and contingent, as they are in Mill's model, but are logical and conceptual. Finally, it should be observed that the concepts in question are open textured; they cannot be defined precisely by reference to a set of necessary and sufficient conditions (Achenstein 1968). The open-textured character of medical concepts may also be used to explain their value dimension; as Kovesi and others have pointed out, one characteristic feature of the open texture of value concepts is that the value component predetermines the selection of criteria for the application of the concept. More attention to this aspect of medical concepts might help us to understand how the elements of particular concepts, for example, the determinants of a particular disease, become a function of their value properties (Kovesi 1967; Brennan 1977).

The value dimensions of these concepts are complicated and multifaceted. Unfortunately, the general attitude of both physicians and laymen towards these questions has often been simplistic and naive. On the one hand, the implicit value dimensions of a particular medical concept are denied and questions of value are put aside and ignored, as if the user were embarrassed to talk about them or did not know what to do with them. On the other hand, values and value claims are embraced uncritically, as if the determination of what has value is simply a matter of subjective feeling and personal (or social) preference. But it should be clear by now that the kind of divorce of values from science that is taken for granted in these attitudes simply lends credence to the applied science model of medicine and to what I have called "medical consumerism." On that account, medicine is no longer concerned with the promotion of health and the prevention and treatment of disease, but simply with supplying a certain kind of medical service demanded by its customers. Like it or not, the value questions implicit in medicine, theoretical as well as practical, cannot be ignored, for to deny them simply amounts to capitulating to prevailing prejudices or interests.[24]

What, then, do we mean by *value*? It is natural to assume that in describing certain medical concepts as value laden, the least that we can mean is that they are connected in some essential way with human purposes and needs or with other important aspects of the human situation. There is nothing wrong with an analysis along these lines, especially as it relates to values in medicine, but we must be careful not to oversimplify the conception of value and to ignore its other facets. We must be prepared to recognize that the connections between values and purposes or needs, as well as connections among values and between values and other things (e.g., actions and attitudes) are not necessarily simple and straightforward. Values, like the other concepts mentioned, are multidimensional: they reach out and connect with many different kinds of things and relate to them in many different kinds of ways. Thus, at one level they connect with human needs and with relevant medical conditions, but at another level, they connect with conduct, feelings, and attitudes.[25] In short, the connections between the concept of value and these other factors are not simple and linear.

VALUES AND ETHICS

One should be careful not to make the mistake of confusing questions of values with questions of ethics. To be sure, values in the sense discussed above constitute one of the considerations to be taken into account in reaching an ethical decision, but questions of ethics do not reduce to questions about values in that sense. Ethics is more closely connected with conduct: with what ought to be done, rather than simply with what is desirable or undesirable apart from any bearing it might have on conduct. But ethics must also take into account factors other than those relating to values; for example, an ethical decision must also be based on a consideration of rights, on previous obligations and prior responsibilities, as well as more general considerations relating to virtues like compassion, honesty, and respect. These more purely ethical considerations characteristically pertain to persons as persons rather than, as values do, to persons as bundles of feelings, needs, purposes, and interests.

THE CRITIQUE OF CONCEPTS

One important function of philosophy is to provide a critical evaluation of concepts, including their interconnections, implications, and presuppositions. We should not assume that values have to be taken at face value, uncriticized. Like other concepts, values often outlive their usefulness and are superseded or restructured. Chastity, which Hume regarded as a virtue in women, has lost its earlier unquestioned value. Bleeding, at one time a highly valued medical treatment, is, for obvious reasons, no longer regarded as such. Scientific, cultural, social, and institutional changes quite properly bring about changes in our concepts and, along with them, changes in our values.

One of the most important, and perhaps most neglected, aspects of the logic of concepts concerns the way in which conceptual connections between the components of a concept are established, broken, or restructured. Chastity and bleeding have lost their value status because the assumptions on which they were based no longer obtain.[27]

To see how covert value considerations are imbedded in medical concepts and how these value connections can be restructured, consider the debate over whether homosexuality and alcoholism are diseases. The use of the concept of disease in connection with alcoholism is intended to break its connection with moral or social disapproval and to establish, instead, a connection with treatment. However, when it is said that homosexuality is not a disease, the intent is to disconnect the connotations that being a homosexual is undesirable and a condition requiring medical treatment.

In addition to these rather obvious examples, there are many other ostensibly descriptive or scientific concepts that contain hidden value implications. Consequently, many debates that appear to be about descriptive or scientific matters are really debates over the values associated with those matters. In order to understand the points at issue, we must make these hidden value implications explicit and then reexamine the validity of the interconnections of the concepts they involve. If we fail to recognize these value aspects of medical concepts or are uncritical of them, we run the risk of being trapped by our own concepts.

The kind of confusion that results from blindness to the value dimensions of concepts is often found in discussions of euthanasia that invoke distinctions such as those between "ordinary" and "extraordinary" measures and between "killing" and "letting die." That there is such a diversity of opinion, even among doctors, over what falls under one of these concepts suggests that the criteria are a function of their value (or ethical) implications rather than the other way around; in other words, their value component determines their content rather than, as is supposed, their content determining their value. Ultimately, these distinctions simply serve as value labels for what a particular person or group regards as an acceptable or unacceptable process. To be specific, what one regards as acceptable in the dying situation one labels as "ordinary" or "letting die," and what one regards as unacceptable one labels "extraordinary" or "killing." Once we see that the substance of the debate over euthanasia is not to be found in these distinctions, which are essentially verbal subterfuges, we will be free to turn our attention to the real medical and ethical issues, which are not nearly as simple and resolvable as an uncritical acceptance of the concepts in question takes for granted that they are. In general, once we become cognizant of the logic of our concepts, we will be better able to cope directly and less mysteriously with the underlying theoretical and practical problems of medicine and society.

These examples show the importance of a critical analytical approach to concepts. Medical discourse provides an abundance of concepts that exhibit features of the kind I have mentioned. A searching analysis of such concepts in all their specificity would appear to be a worthwhile, if not urgently necessary, task. It is a task on which philosophy and medicine can work together in their common pursuit of a deeper understanding of the nature and role of medicine and its place in modern life.

Notes

1. There are writers who have written on subjects touching on philosophy of medicine, but there is no major philosopher who has had the kind of interest in medicine that Descartes, Leibniz, and Kant, for example, had in mathematics, physics, or astronomy.

2. It is interesting to note in this regard that half of the "best known rabbinical scholars and authors in medieval times were physicians by occupation" (Jakobovits 1978, 2:791). It is no accident, therefore, that the bulk of writings in medical ethics are by persons with a theological background.

3. If it is a science, it is hard to see how medicine would need to appeal to "miracle, mystery, and authority."

4. For the sake of exposition, I have slightly altered the order of the sentences.

5. In my view, conceptual analysis is not a modern invention, but is the method that philosophers have used since the time of Socrates and Plato. It includes, of course, the kinds of analyses found in Descartes, Hume, and Kant. Popular criticism of contemporary analytical philosophy is often justified, not on the grounds that it is analytical, but because it has concerned itself with trivial matters and has often led to trivial results. Philosophy of medicine, I argue, is not trivial in either of these two respects.

6. Kant says that it is *zetetic*, that is, a "searching"; the continuous inquiry after truth.

7. The concept to be analyzed is usually referred to as the *analysandum* and the concept or set of concepts used to analyze is referred to as the *analysans*.

8. On this view, a philosophical analysis is required to preserve the truth values of the original analysandum in the new analysans. The preservation of truth value equivalence is assumed to be a necessary condition of a satisfactory analysis.

9. The passive conception of analysis is the preferred philosophical method in certain branches of philosophy, for example, epistemology. As I hope to make clear, it is not for the most part suitable in ethics and other branches of practical philosophy, and perhaps also not in philosophy of science.

10. I have argued this point more extensively as it relates to ethics in my essay, "The Interdependence of Ethical Analysis and Ethics" (1973).

11. With apologies to Marx! It should be observed that the failure to respond to the activist's challenge simply amounts to an intellectual acceptance of the status quo.

12. One reason why philosophers have paid so little attention in the past to subjects like medicine is that they have failed to appreciate the philosophical importance of the network of conceptual problems connected with the relationship between scientific theory and social practice in general, that is, there has been no interest in developing a philosophy of technology.

13. See *Nicomachean Ethics*, book VI, especially chapter 4. There are references to the concept of *technē* in many other writings of Aristotle, but it is unnecessary to examine them here.

14. The feature that both types of reasoning have in common is that they involve some kind of expertise and they can be taught.

15. These comparisons may be found in a number of passages in the *Nicomachean Ethics*, the *Metaphysics*, and the *Politics*.

16. Terence Irwin has some interesting comments on this aspect of *technē* in Plato, who, in the Socratic dialogues, appears to accept the view that moral virtue is a kind of *technē* (1977, pp. 71ff). There are similarities and dissimilarities in detail between the conceptions of *technē* held by Socrates, Plato, and Aristotle.

17. It might also be called the technological model.

18. The ends of technological medicine are also, of course, determined by economic interests, for example, of the physician, of the hospital, of a drug company, or even of the state.

19. A full defense of this thesis is beyond the scope of this essay. A careful study of some of the literature relating to such topics as the logic of clinical diagnosis might provide arguments that could be used to support the contention that the positivistic principles in question imply that many if not most accepted diagnostic techniques are unscientific!

20. See, for example, the discussions of disease classification and their relationship to prediction and treatment in Wulff (1976).

21. One simple example of how value considerations creep into science is pointed out by Leach in an article on the assessment of evidence and acceptable error. Obviously, in medicine the criteria of an acceptable hypothesis are connected with "pragmatic utilities" (1974, pp. 466-83).

22. The notion of a logic of scientific discovery was first suggested by N.R. Hanson in his *Patterns of Discovery* (1958). For a useful discussion, see Hanson (1961).

23. The issues involved here are discussed in more detail by Stephen Toulmin (1985).

24. Ivan Illich (1975) has pointed out some of these aspects of medicine in a rather extreme way. However, I think that Illich misses the point that I have been making here, namely, that for good or bad, the value problems

in modern medicine are bound up logically with the conceptual apparatus and framework of medical thought. In that sense, Illich's teaching is rhetorical rather than analytical or critical.

25. These aspects of the concept of value have been discussed extensively in the philosophical literature on the subject.

26. Actions or decisions often require choosing between alternatives. In such cases, ethics must select between values and reflect on what ought to be done, not on the basis of a single value, but on a comparative assessment of competing values.

27. Hume based his argument that chastity is a virtue on the premise that if a woman is not chaste, she will become pregnant. Apart from all the other reasons for rejecting Hume's doctrine, it is sufficient to point out that in today's world, pregnancy is not the inevitable result of sexual intercourse. (See Hume 1888, book iii, part ii, sec. xii).

Bibliography

Achinstein, P. 1968. *Concepts of Science*. Baltimore: Johns Hopkins Press.

Brennan, J.M. 1977. *The Open Texture of Moral Concepts*. New York: Barnes and Noble.

Cassirer, E., ed. 1912. *Immanuel Kants Werke*. Berlin: Bruno Cassirer.

Feinstein, A. 1973. "An Analysis of Diagnostic Reasoning." *Yale Journal of Biology and Medicine* 46: 212-32.

_____ . 1974. "An Analysis of Diagnostic Reasoning." *Yale Journal of Biology and Medicine* 47: 5-32.

Gorovitz, S. and MacIntyre, A. 1976. "Toward a Theory of Medical Fallibility." In *Science, Ethics and Medicine*, edited by H.T. Engelhardt, Jr. and D. Callahan. Hastings-on-Hudson, NY: The Hastings Center.

Hanson, N.R. 1958. *Patterns of Discovery*. London: Cambridge University Press.

_____ . 1961. "Is There a Logic of Scientific Discovery?" In *Current Issues in the Philosophy of Science*, edited by H. Feigl and C. Maxwell. New York: Holt, Rinehart and Winston.

Hempel, C.G. 1968. *Philosophy of Natural Science*. Englewood Cliffs, NJ: Prentice-Hall.

Hull, D. 1974. *Philosophy of Biological Science*. Englewood Cliffs, NJ: Prentice-Hall.

Hume, D. 1888. *Treatise of Human Nature*, edited by L.A. Selby-Bigge. Oxford: Clarendon Press.

Illich, I. 1975. *Medical Nemesis*. New York: Random House.

Irwin, T. 1977. *Plato's Moral Theory*. Oxford: Clarendon Press.

Jakobovits, I. 1978. "Judaism." In *Encyclopedia of Bioethics*, edited by W.T. Reich. New York: Free Press.

Kovesi, J. 1967. *Moral Notions*. New York: Humanities Press.

Ladd, J. 1973. "The Interdependence of Ethical Analysis and Ethics." In *Etyka II*. Warsaw.

Leach, J. 1974. "Explanation and Value Neutrality." In *Philosophical Problems in Science and Technology,* edited by A.C. Michalos. Boston: Allyn and Bacon.

Mill, J.S. 1872. *A System of Logic.* New York: Harper and Brothers.

Toulmin, S. 1985. "Causation and the Locus of Medical Intervention," pp. 59-72 in this volume.

Wittgenstein, L. 1961. *Tractatus Logico-Philosophicus,* translated by D.F. Pears and B.F. McGuiness. London: Routledge and Kegan Paul.

Wulff, H.R. 1976. *Rational Diagnosis and Treatment.* Oxford: Blackwell Scientific Publications.